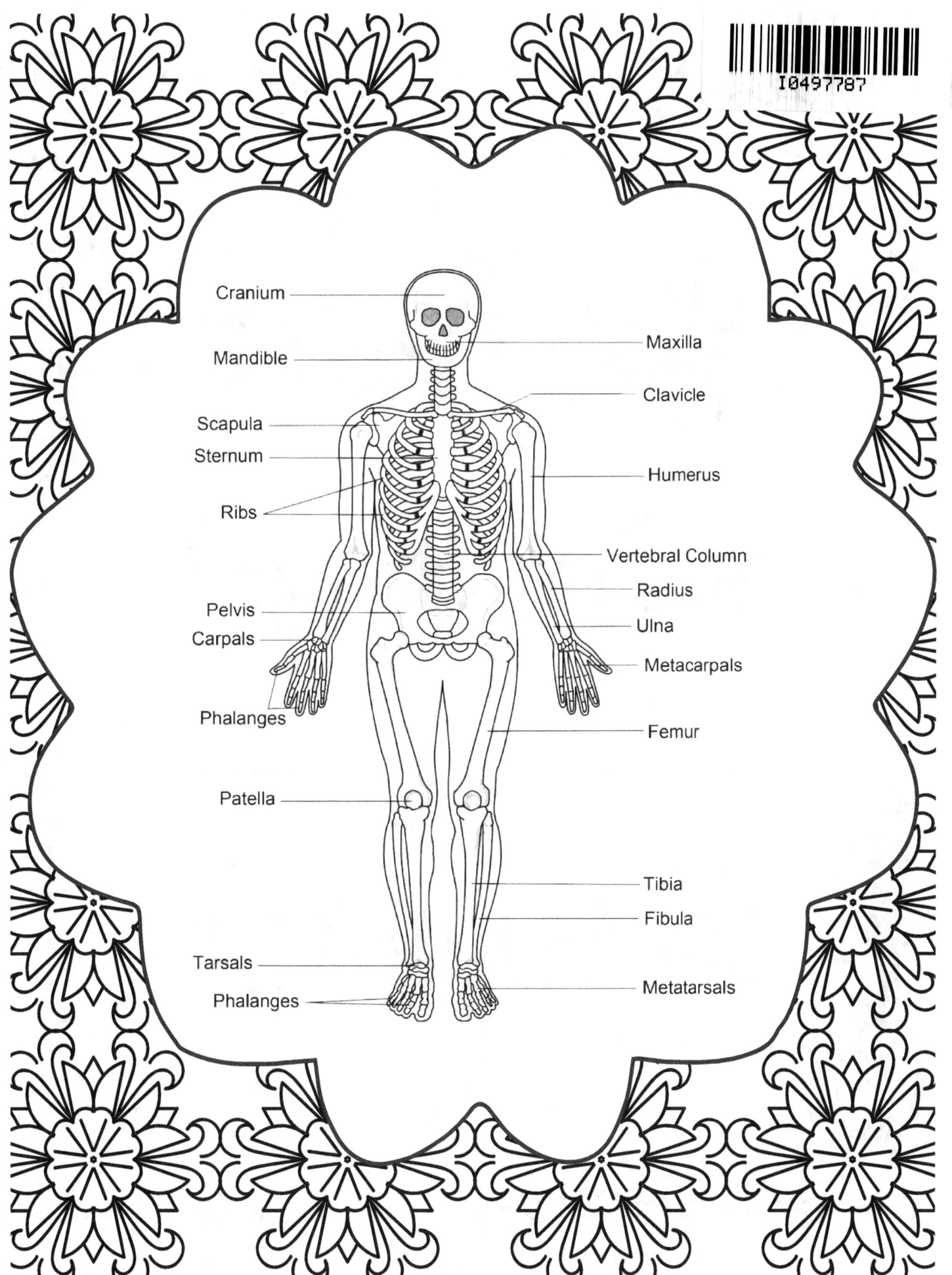

This Book Belongs To

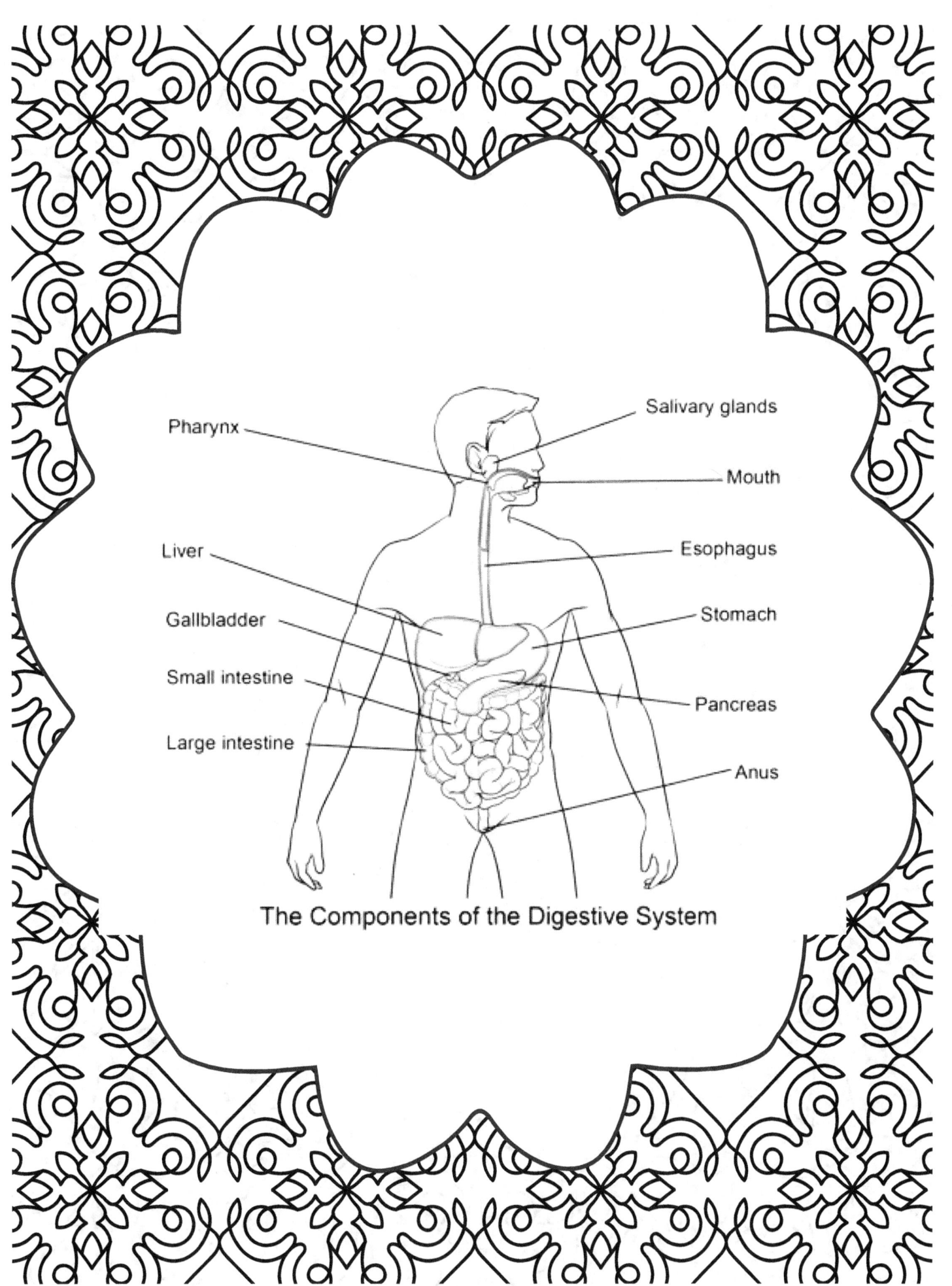

The Components of the Digestive System

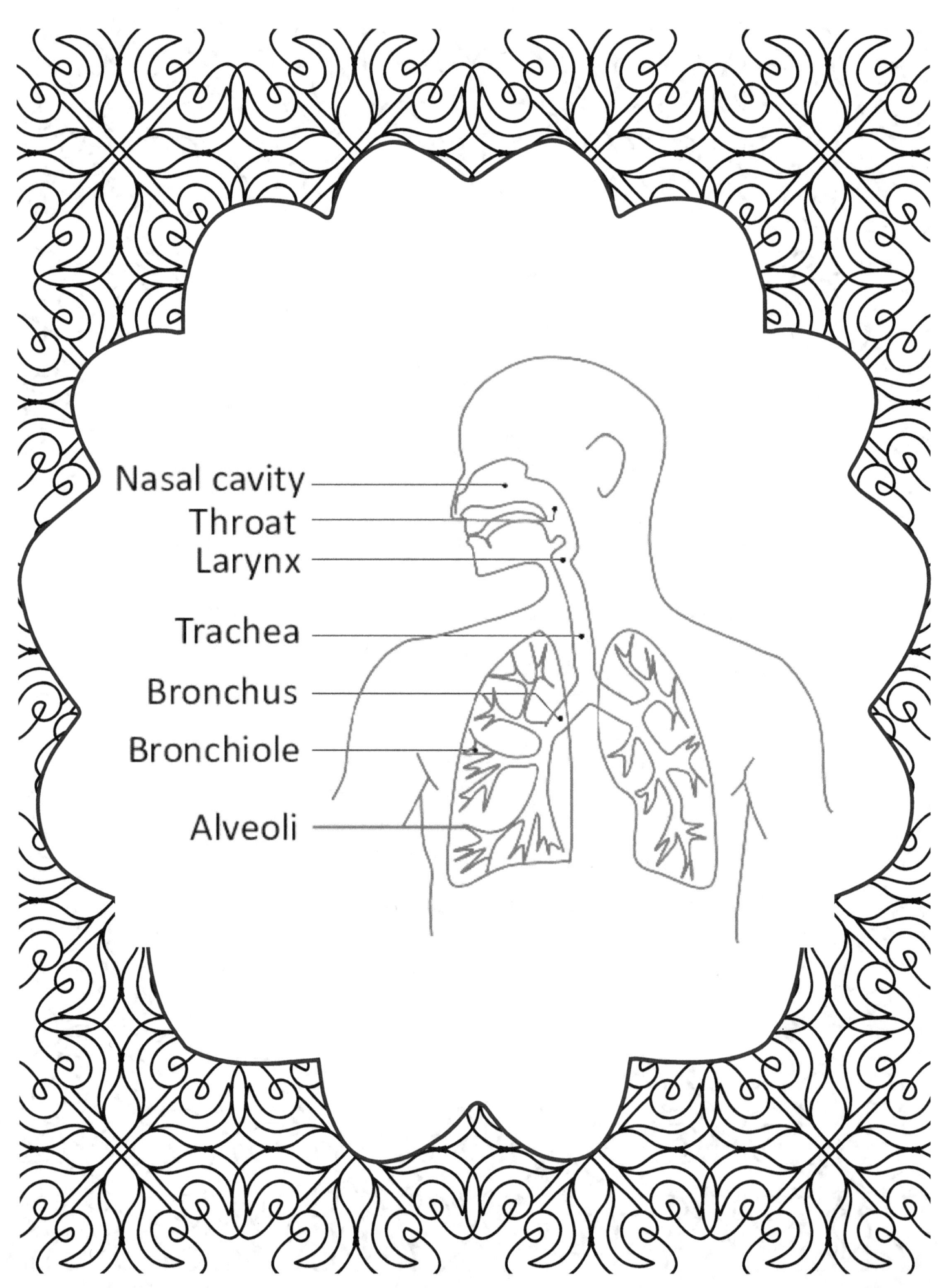

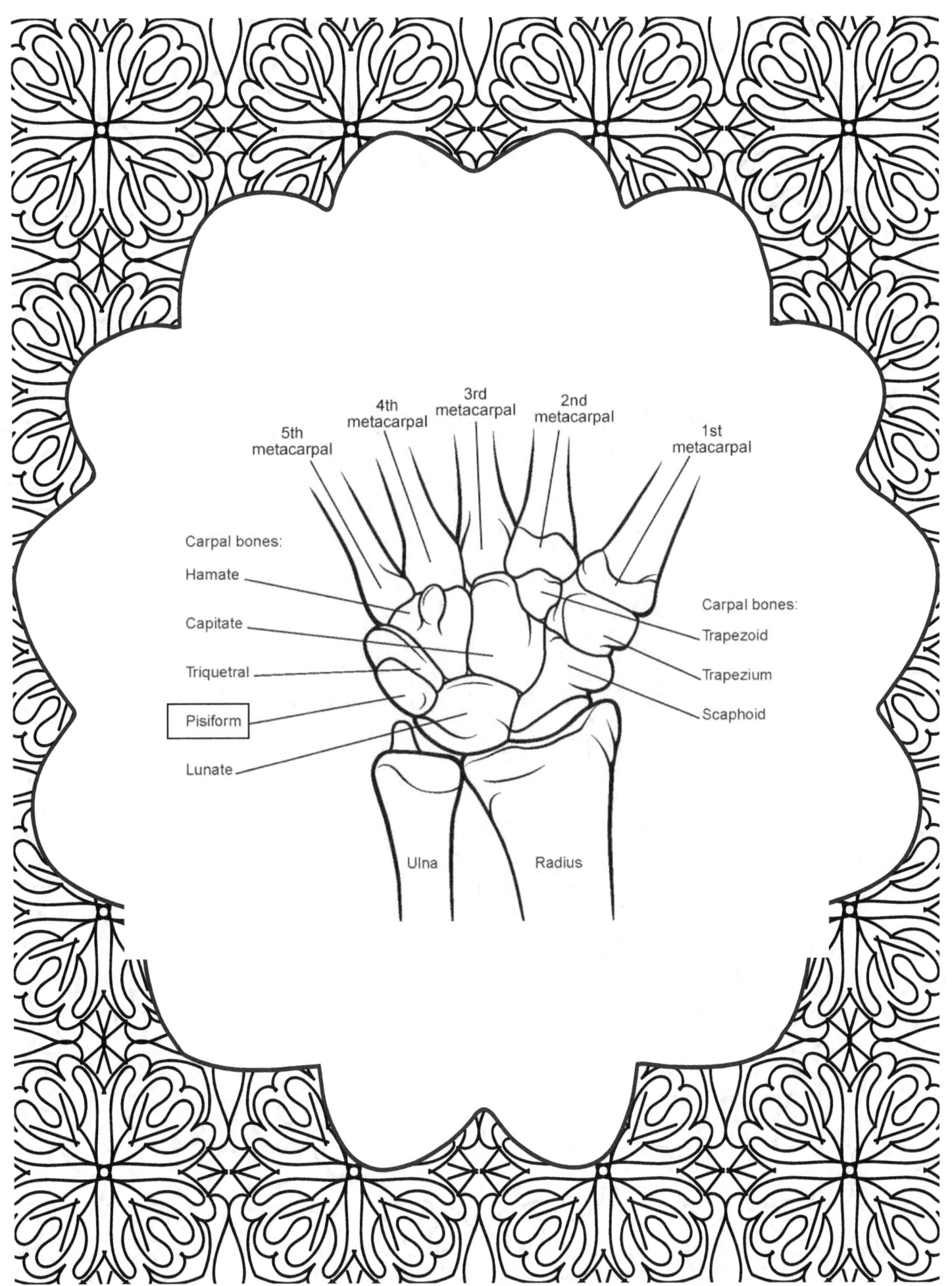

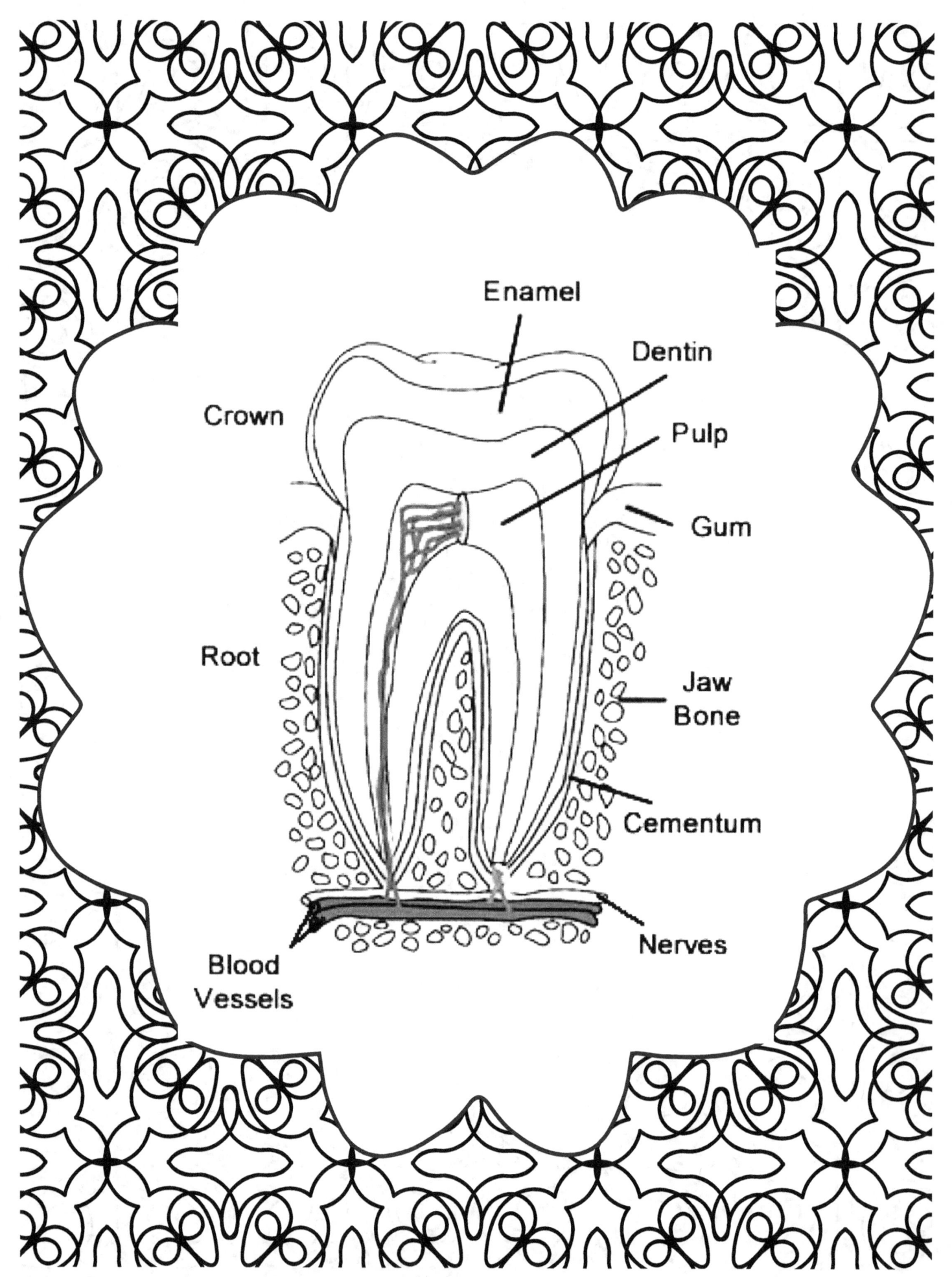

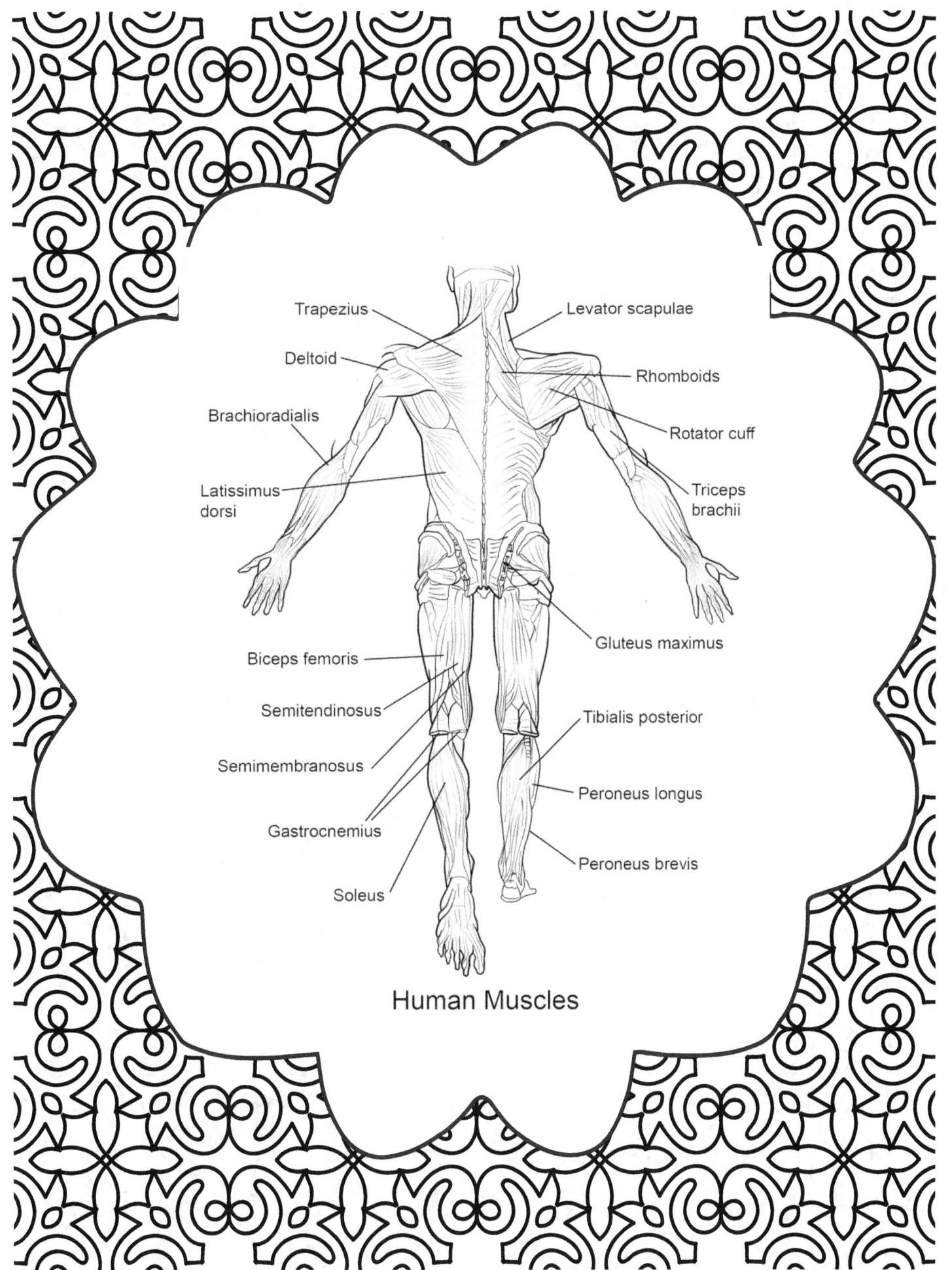

Human Muscles

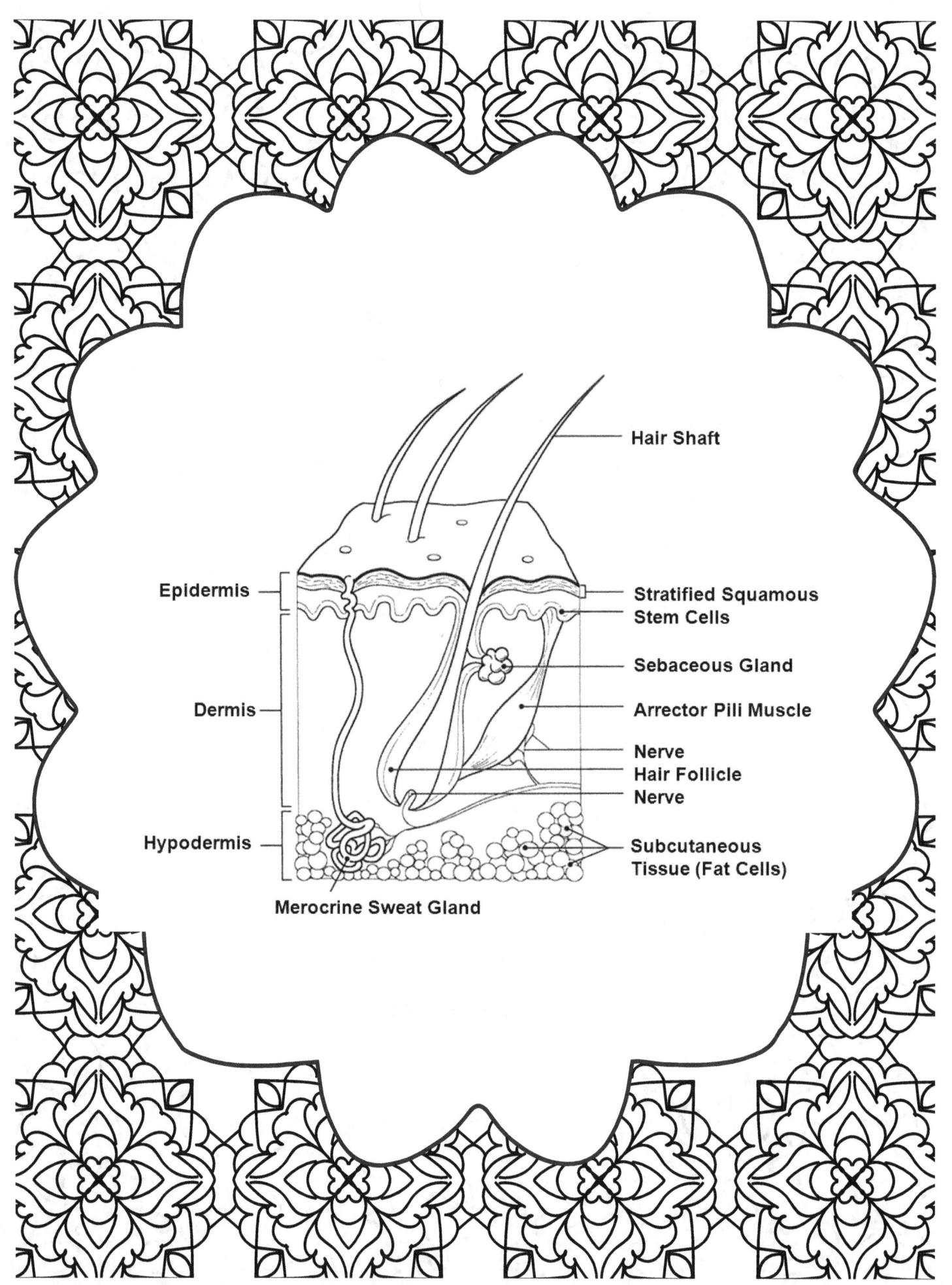

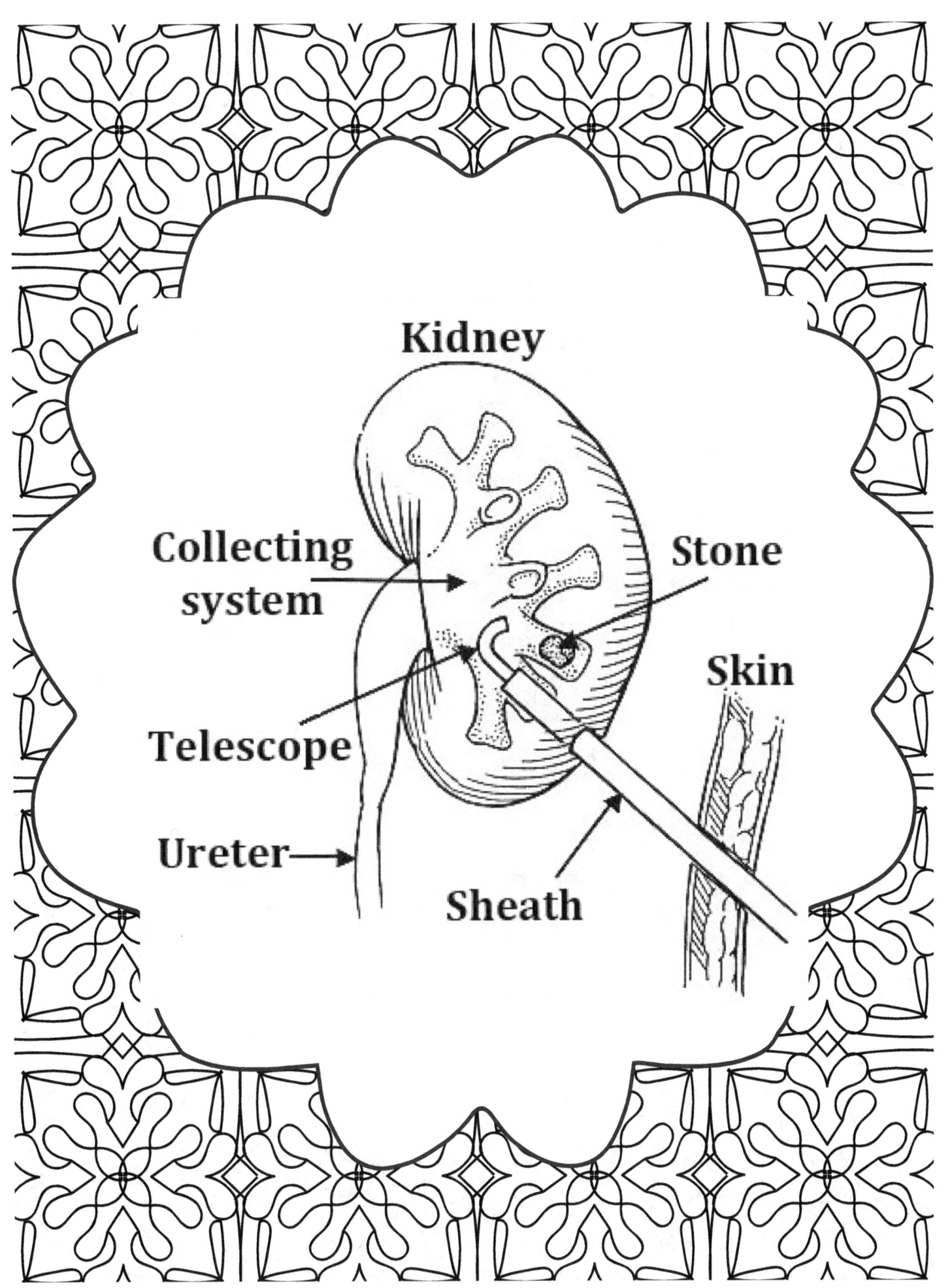

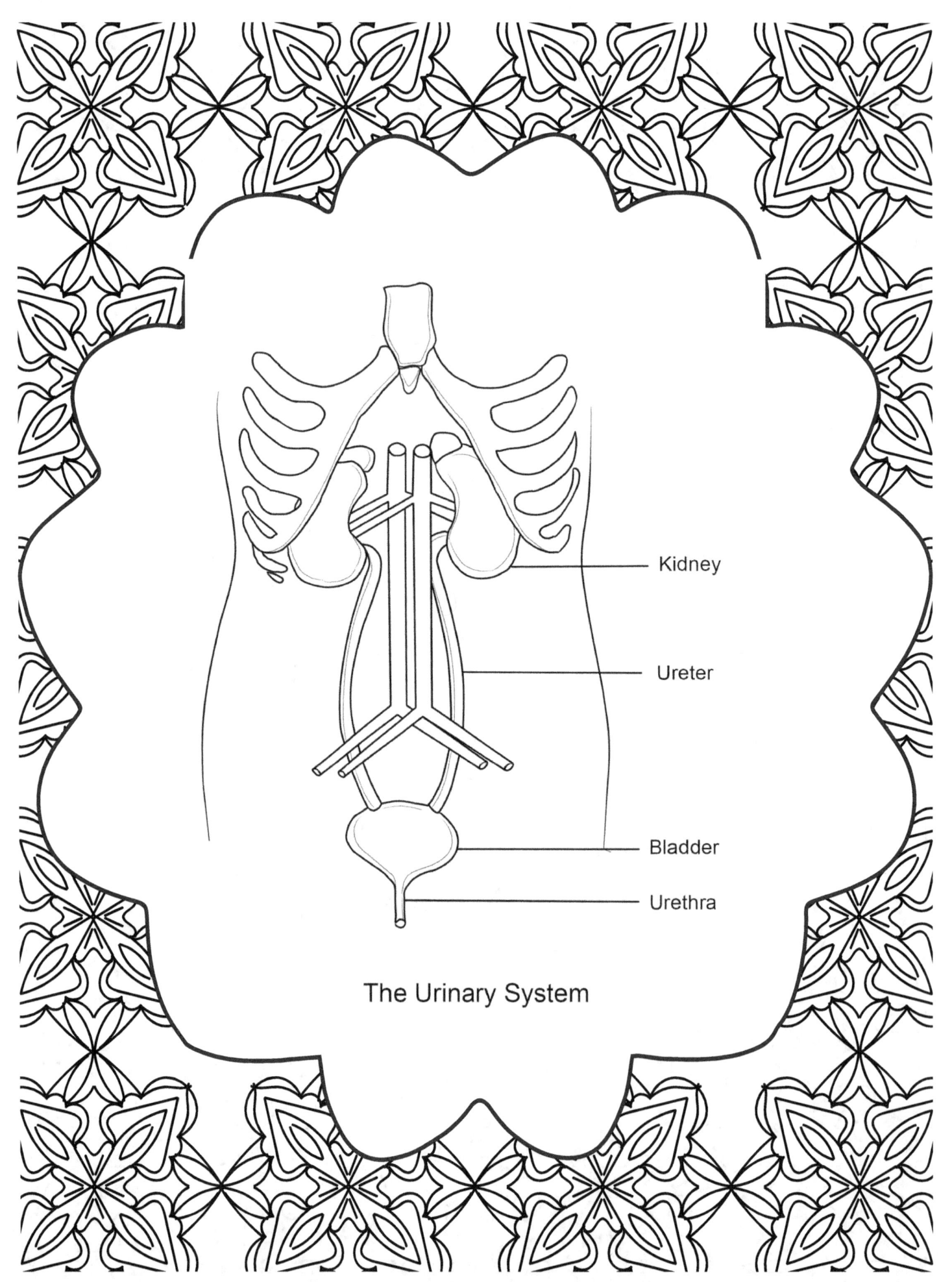

Kidney

Ureter

Bladder

Urethra

The Urinary System

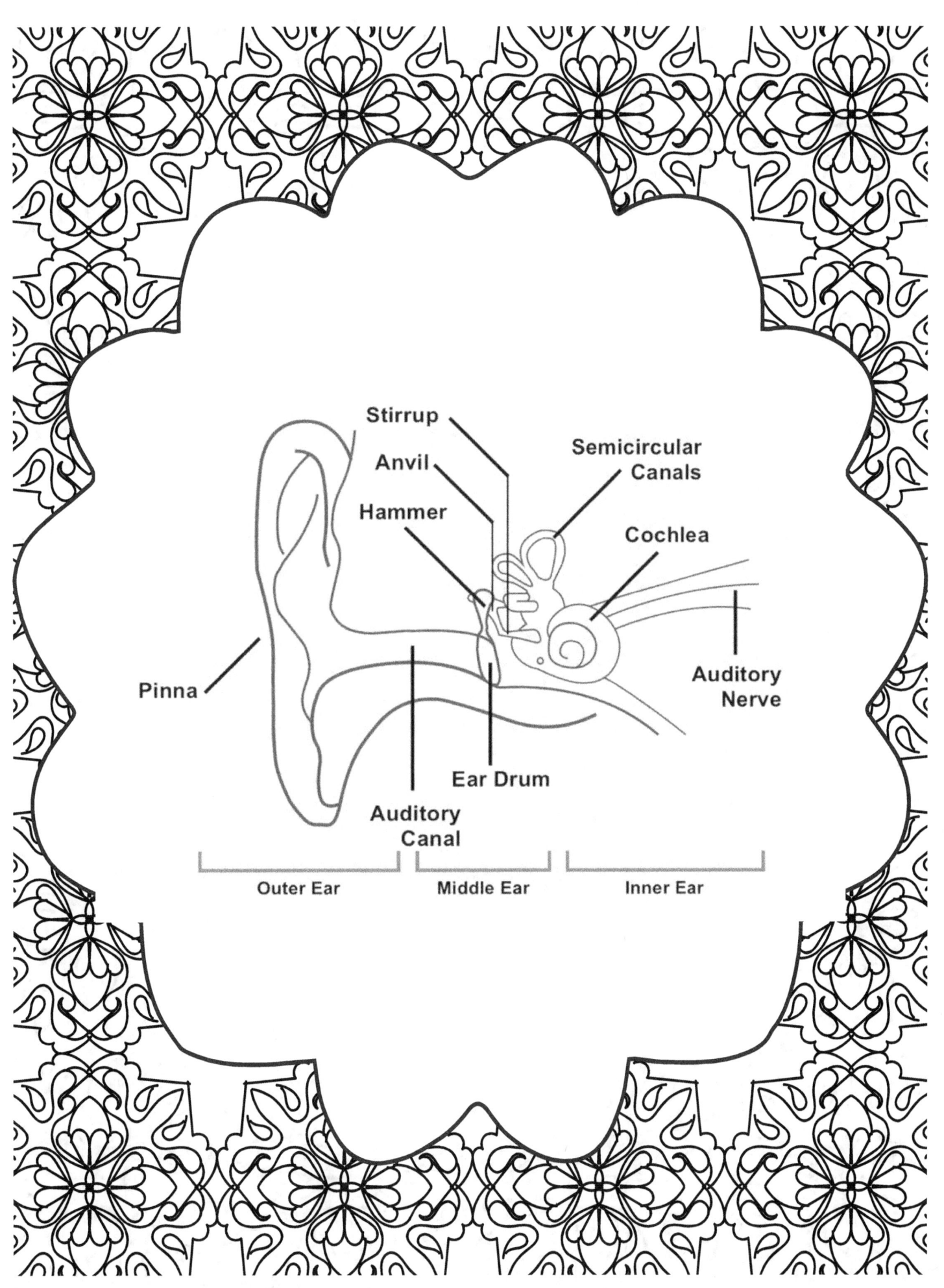

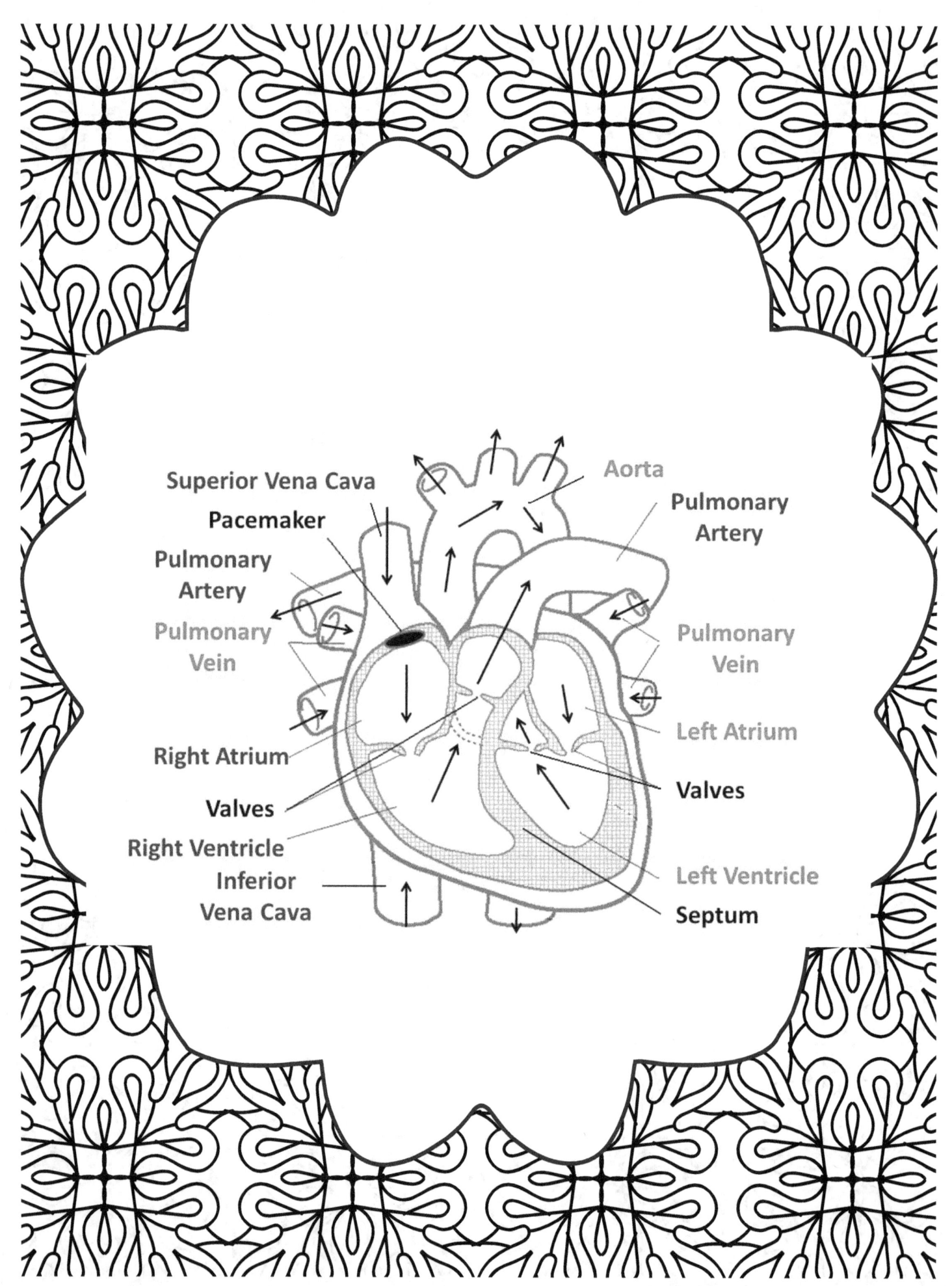

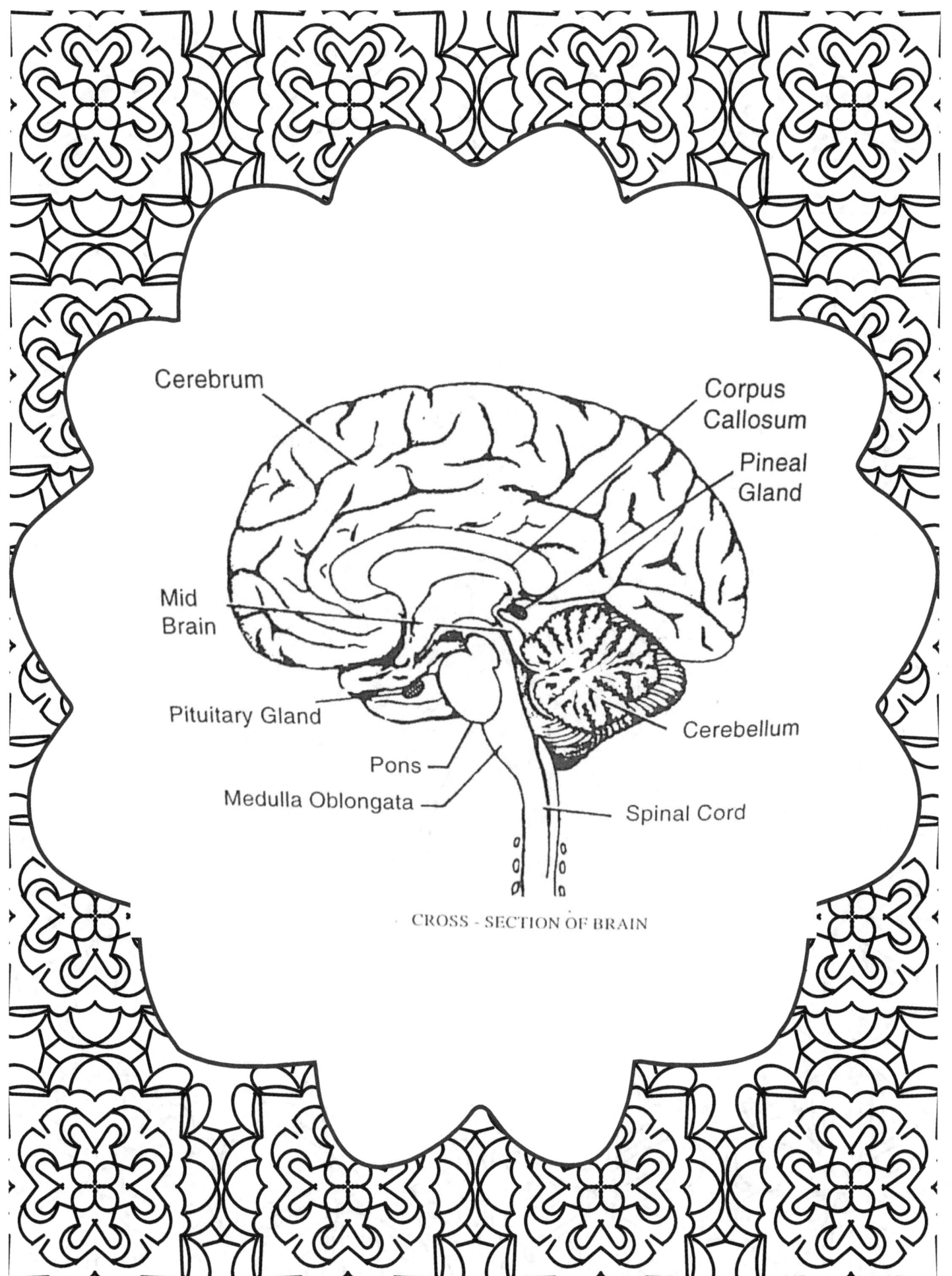

Cerebrum

Corpus Callosum

Pineal Gland

Mid Brain

Pituitary Gland

Cerebellum

Pons

Medulla Oblongata

Spinal Cord

CROSS - SECTION OF BRAIN

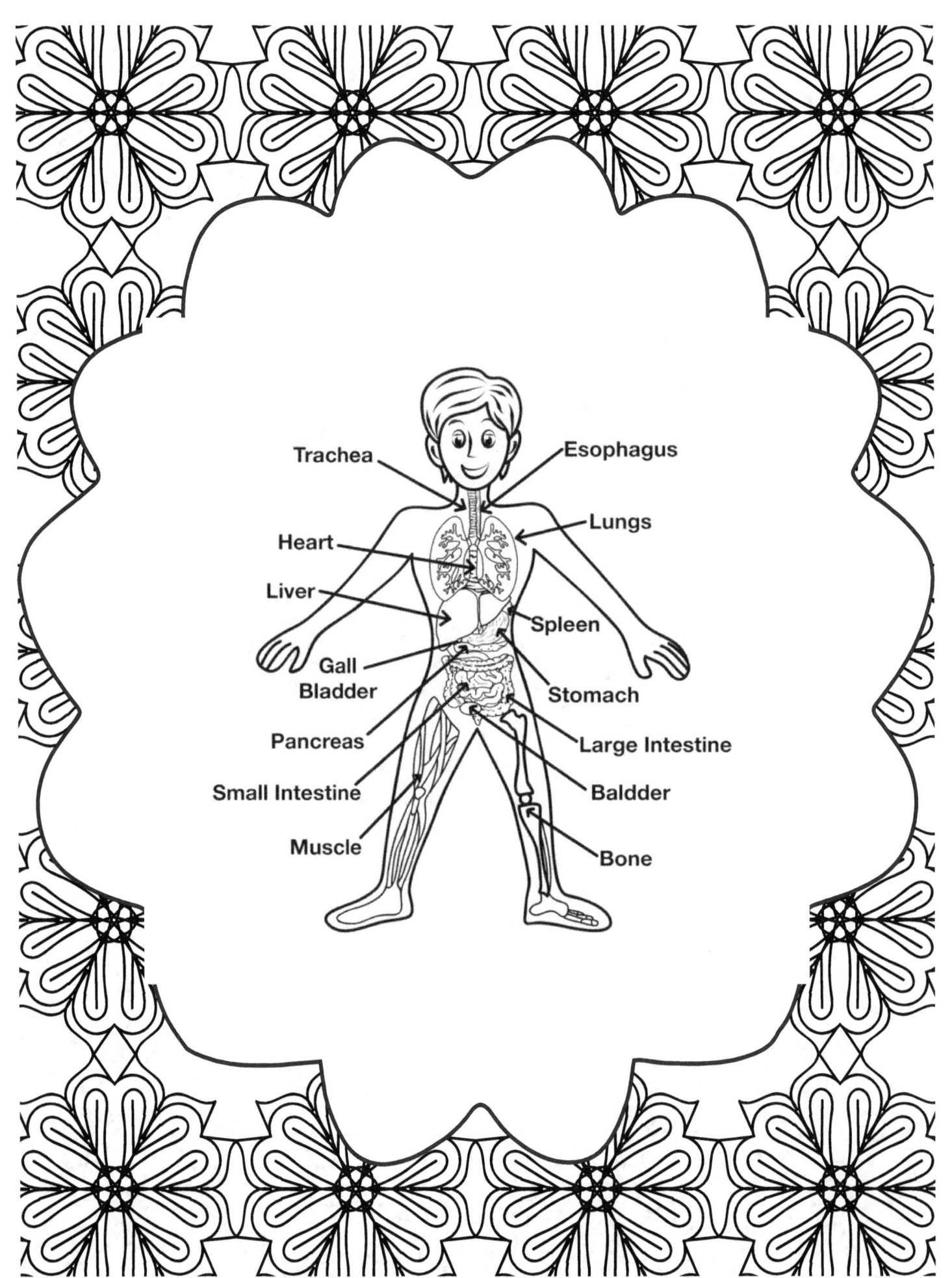

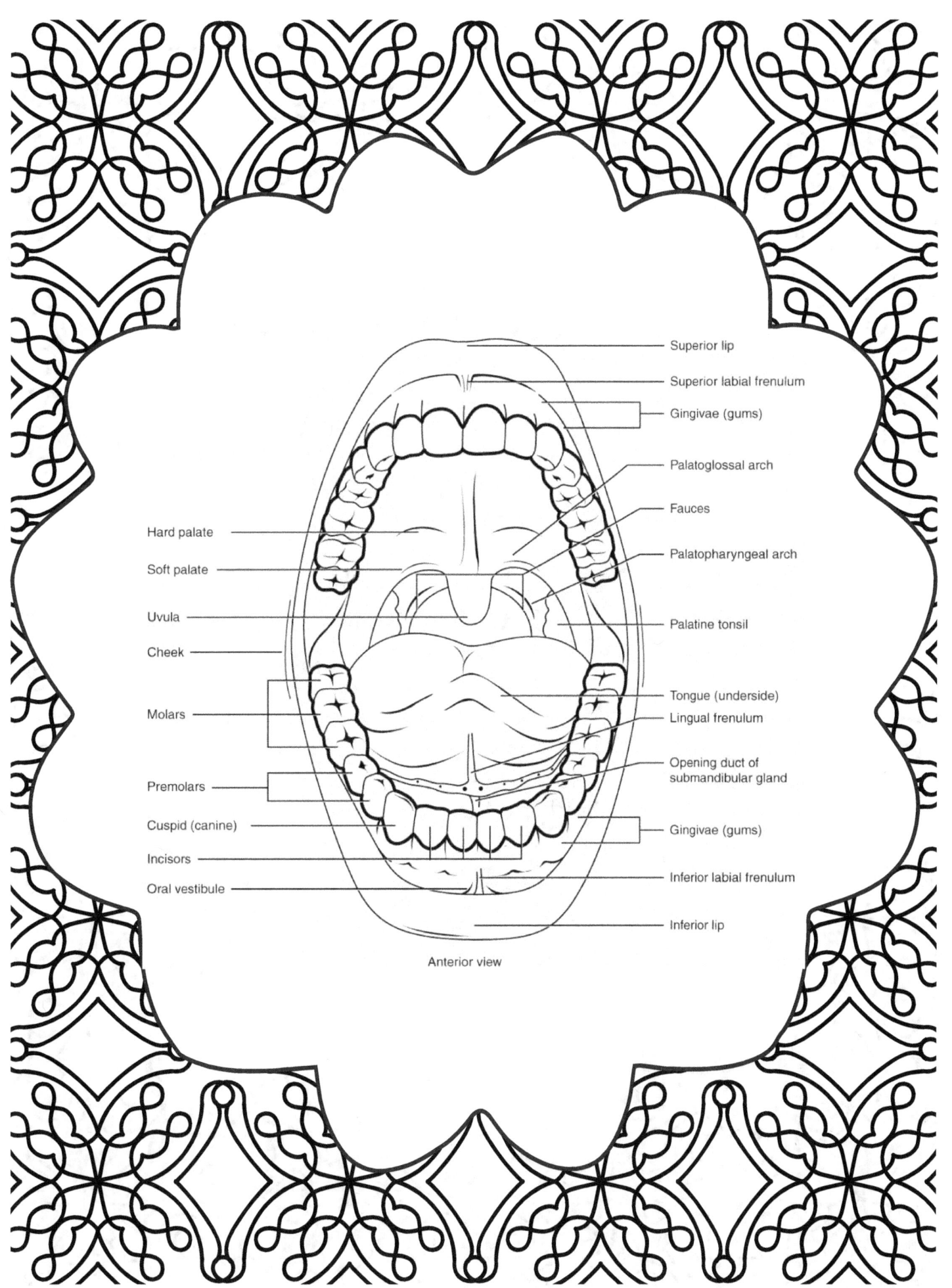

Superior lip

Superior labial frenulum

Gingivae (gums)

Palatoglossal arch

Fauces

Palatopharyngeal arch

Palatine tonsil

Tongue (underside)

Lingual frenulum

Opening duct of
submandibular gland

Gingivae (gums)

Inferior labial frenulum

Inferior lip

Hard palate

Soft palate

Uvula

Cheek

Molars

Premolars

Cuspid (canine)

Incisors

Oral vestibule

Anterior view

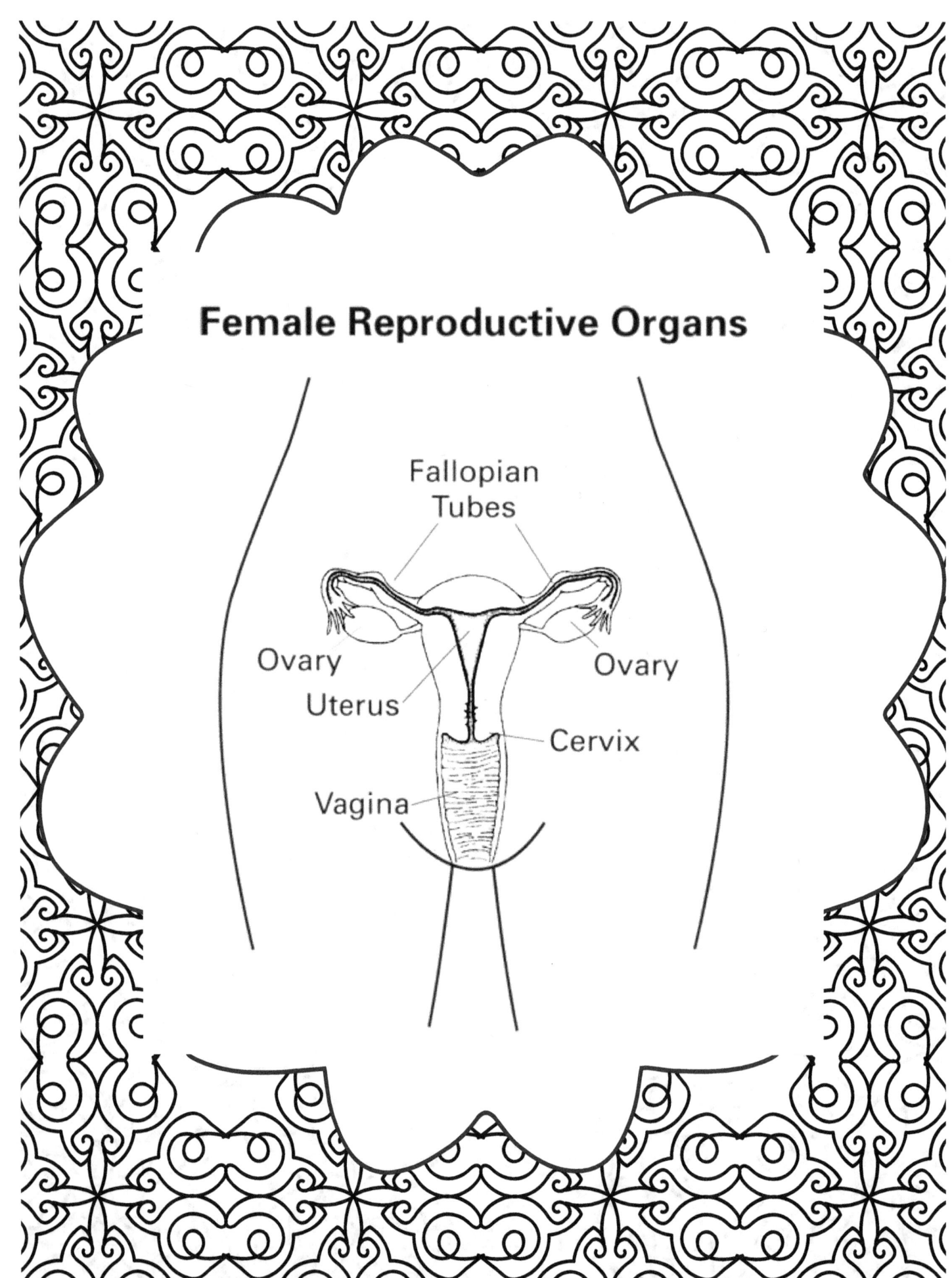

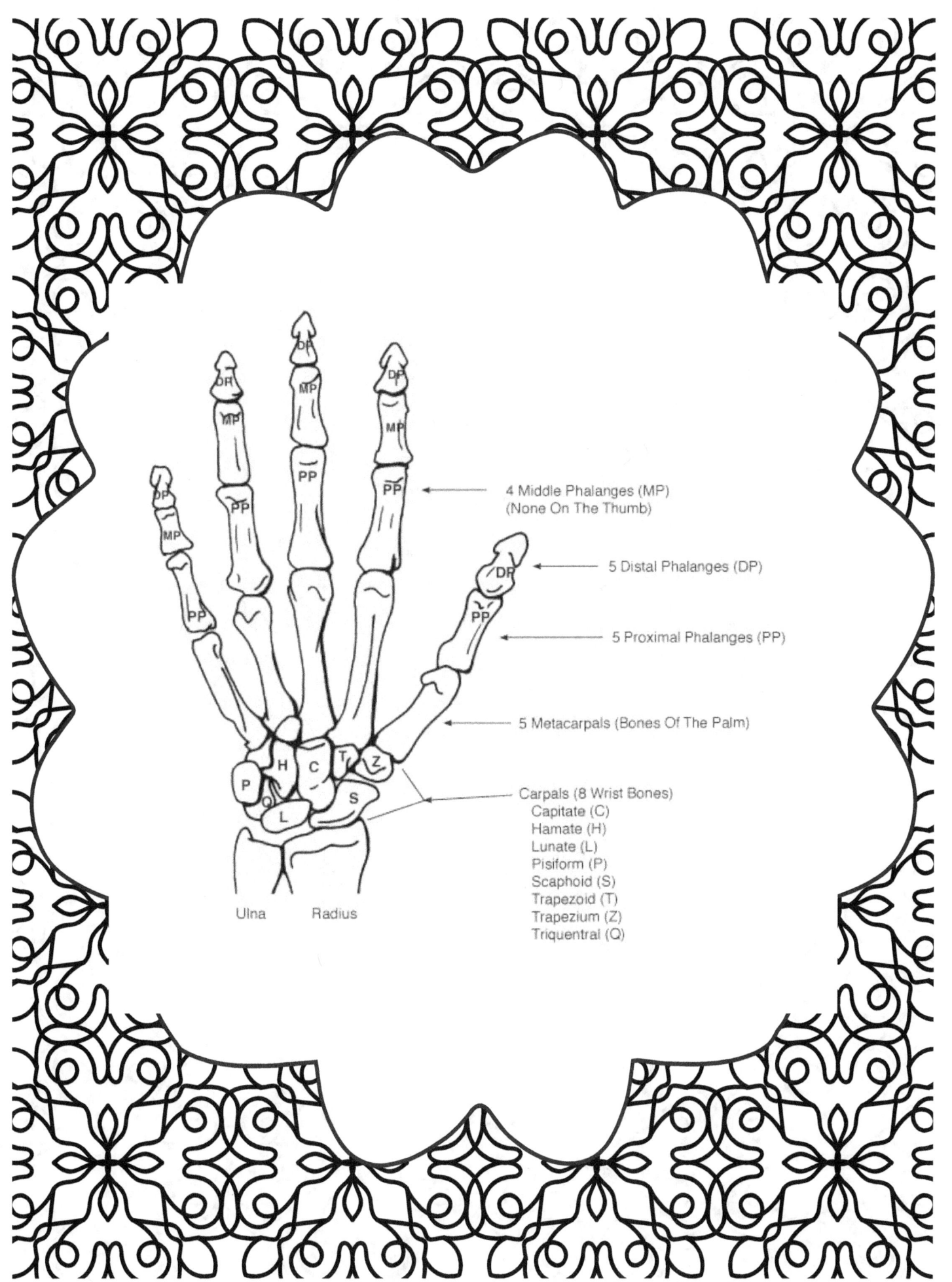

4 Middle Phalanges (MP)
(None On The Thumb)

5 Distal Phalanges (DP)

5 Proximal Phalanges (PP)

5 Metacarpals (Bones Of The Palm)

Carpals (8 Wrist Bones)
   Capitate (C)
   Hamate (H)
   Lunate (L)
   Pisiform (P)
   Scaphoid (S)
   Trapezoid (T)
   Trapezium (Z)
   Triquentral (Q)

Ulna   Radius

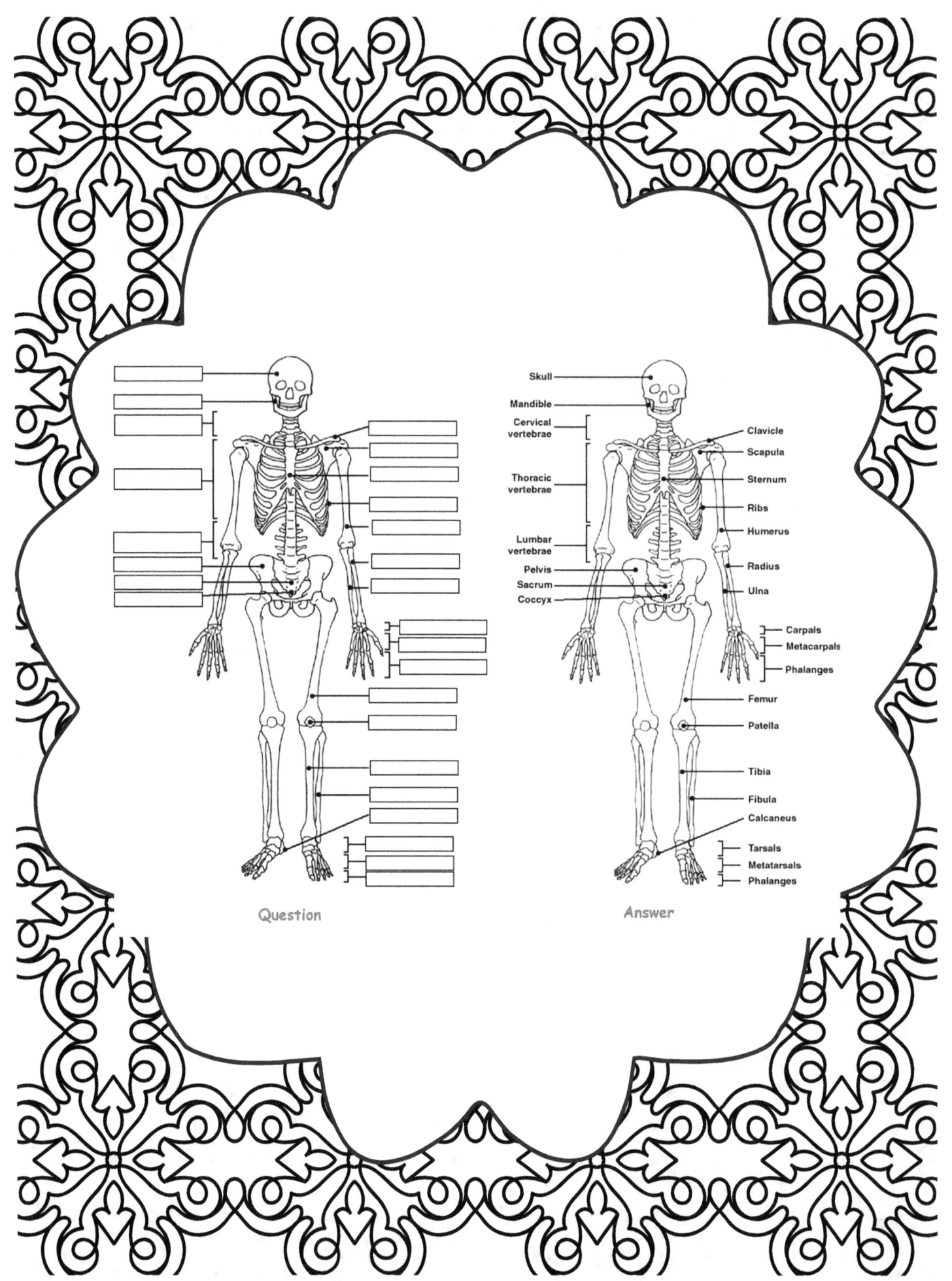

Question

Answer

Skull
Mandible
Cervical vertebrae
Thoracic vertebrae
Lumbar vertebrae
Pelvis
Sacrum
Coccyx
Clavicle
Scapula
Sternum
Ribs
Humerus
Radius
Ulna
Carpals
Metacarpals
Phalanges
Femur
Patella
Tibia
Fibula
Calcaneus
Tarsals
Metatarsals
Phalanges

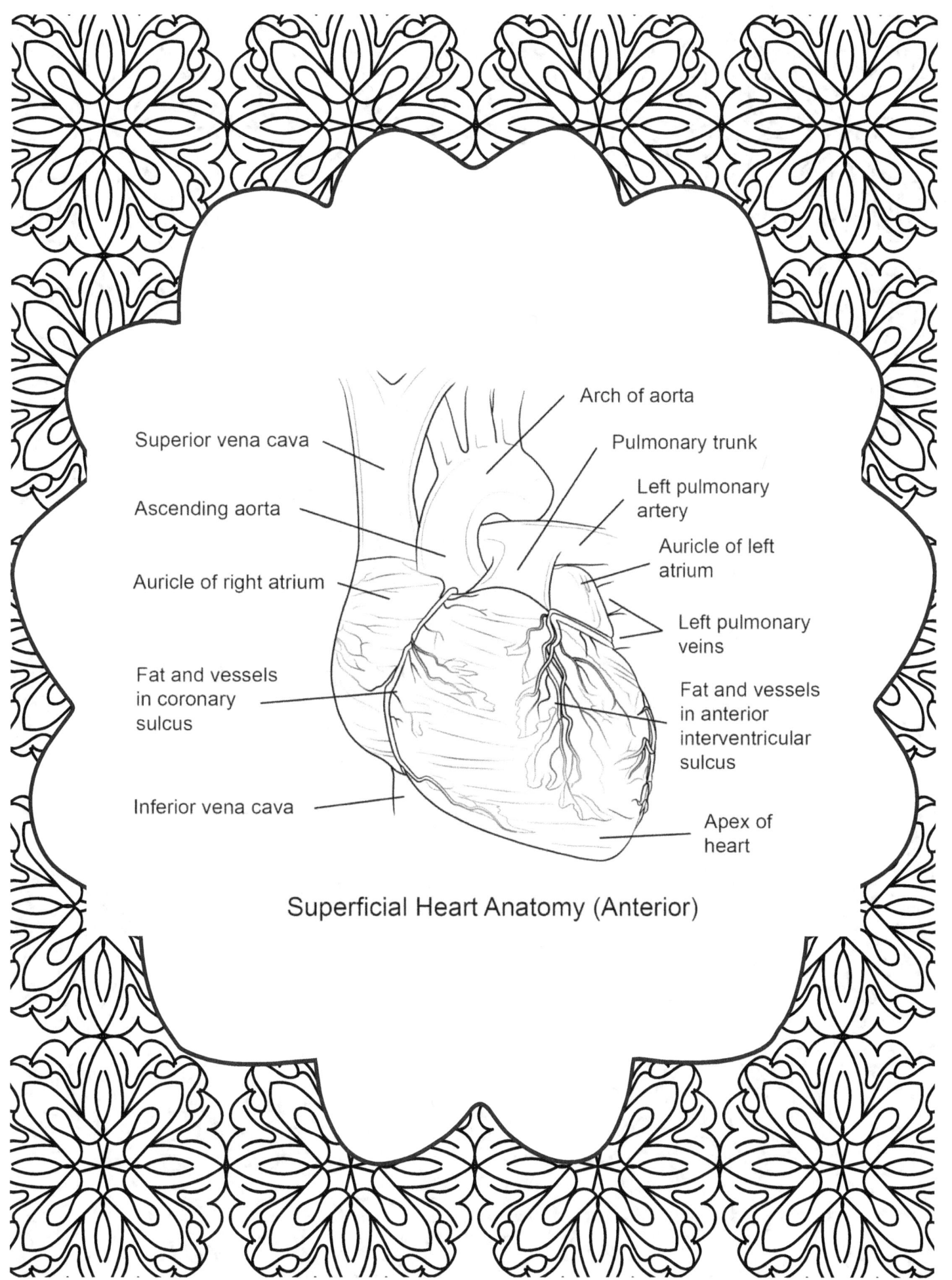

Arch of aorta

Superior vena cava

Pulmonary trunk

Ascending aorta

Left pulmonary artery

Auricle of left atrium

Auricle of right atrium

Left pulmonary veins

Fat and vessels in coronary sulcus

Fat and vessels in anterior interventricular sulcus

Inferior vena cava

Apex of heart

Superficial Heart Anatomy (Anterior)

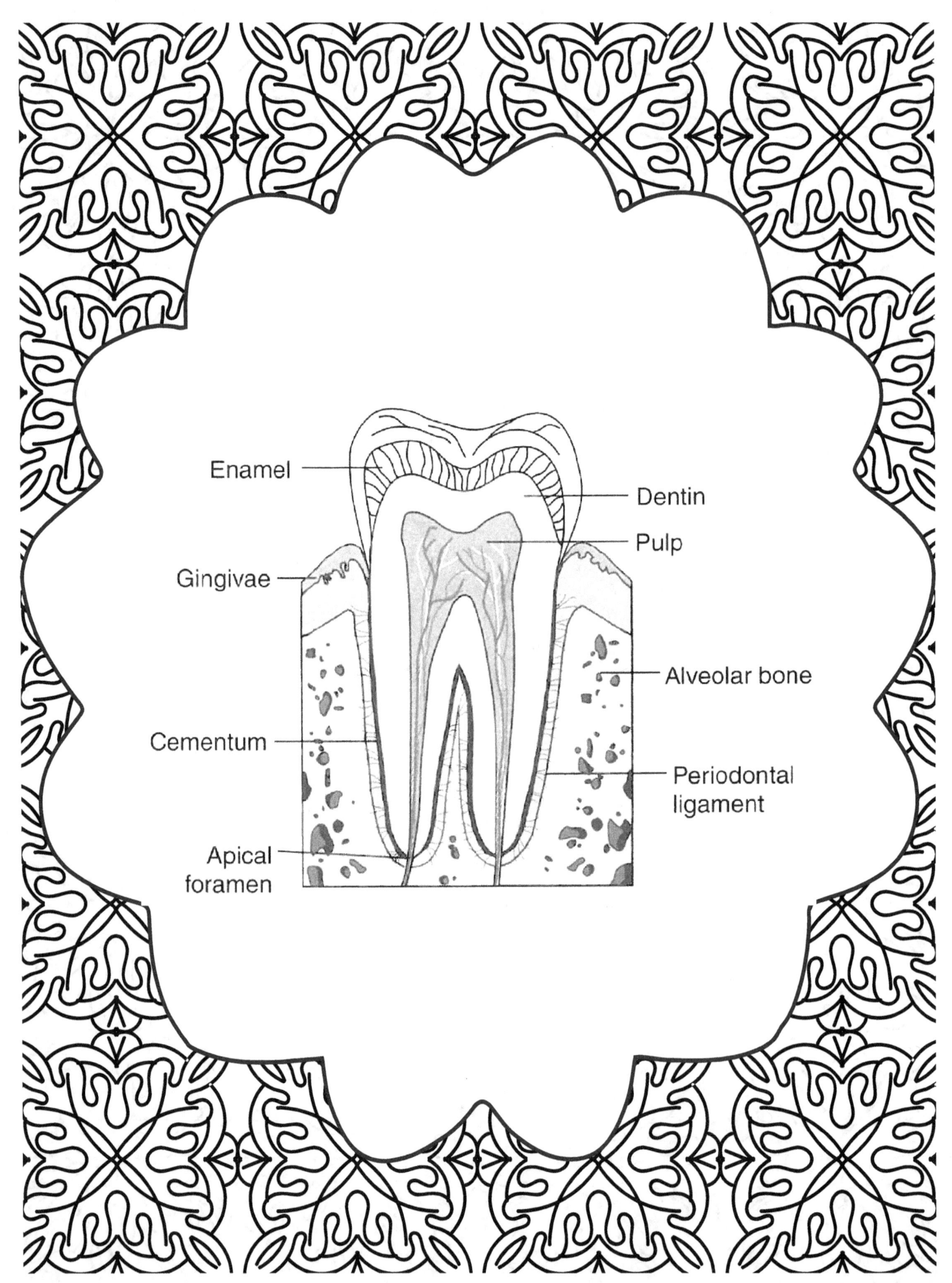

parts of an ear

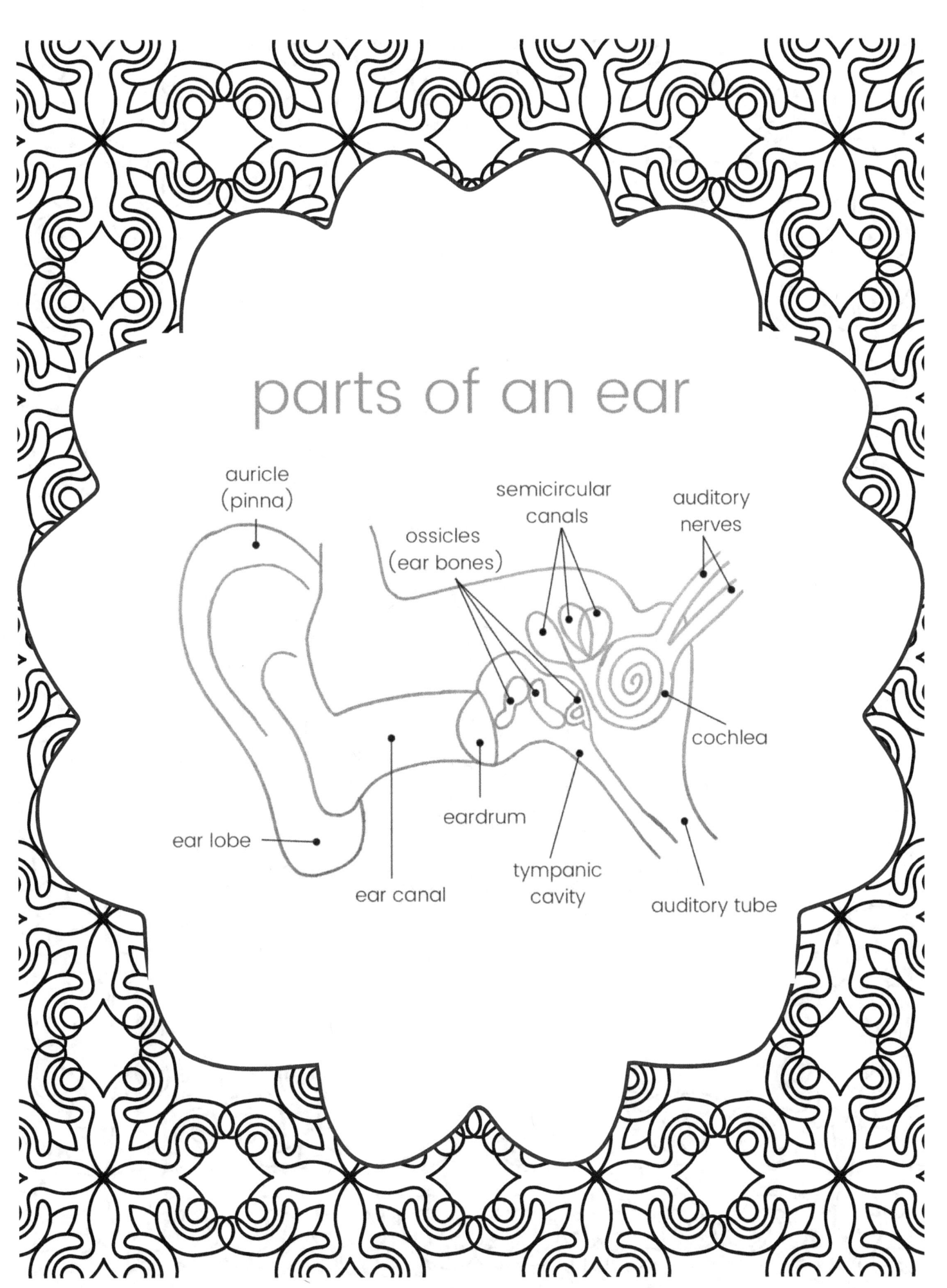

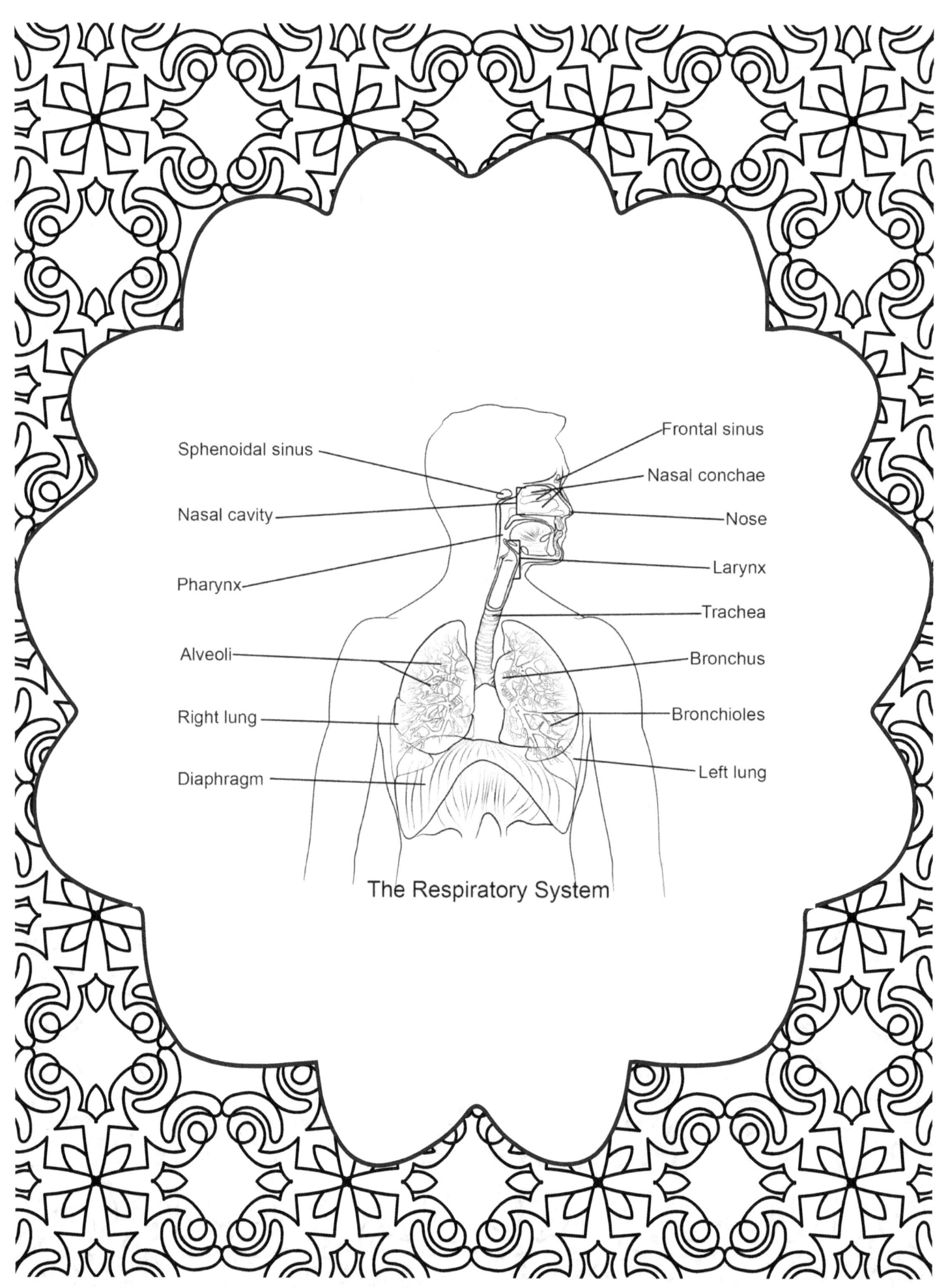

The Respiratory System

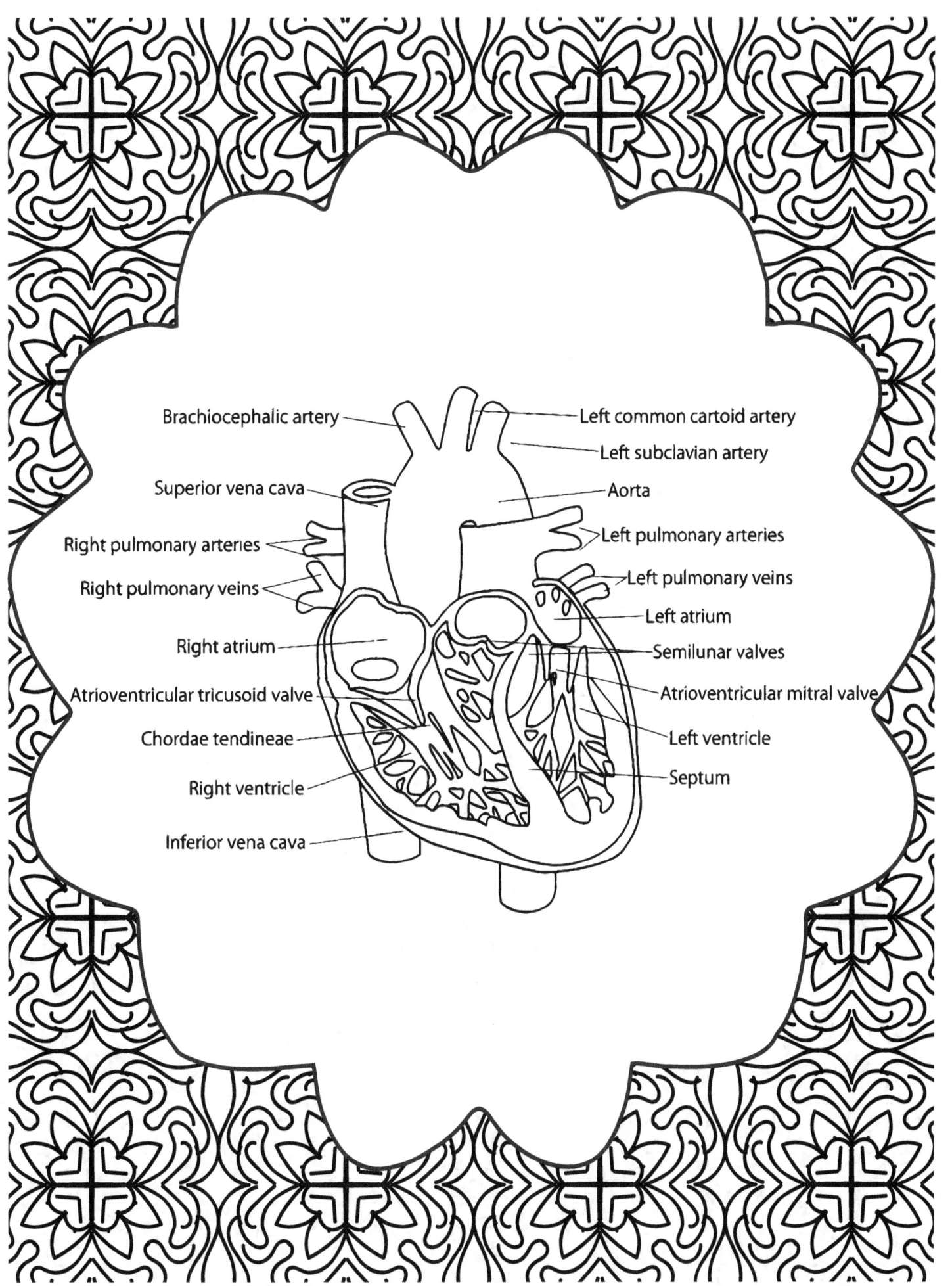

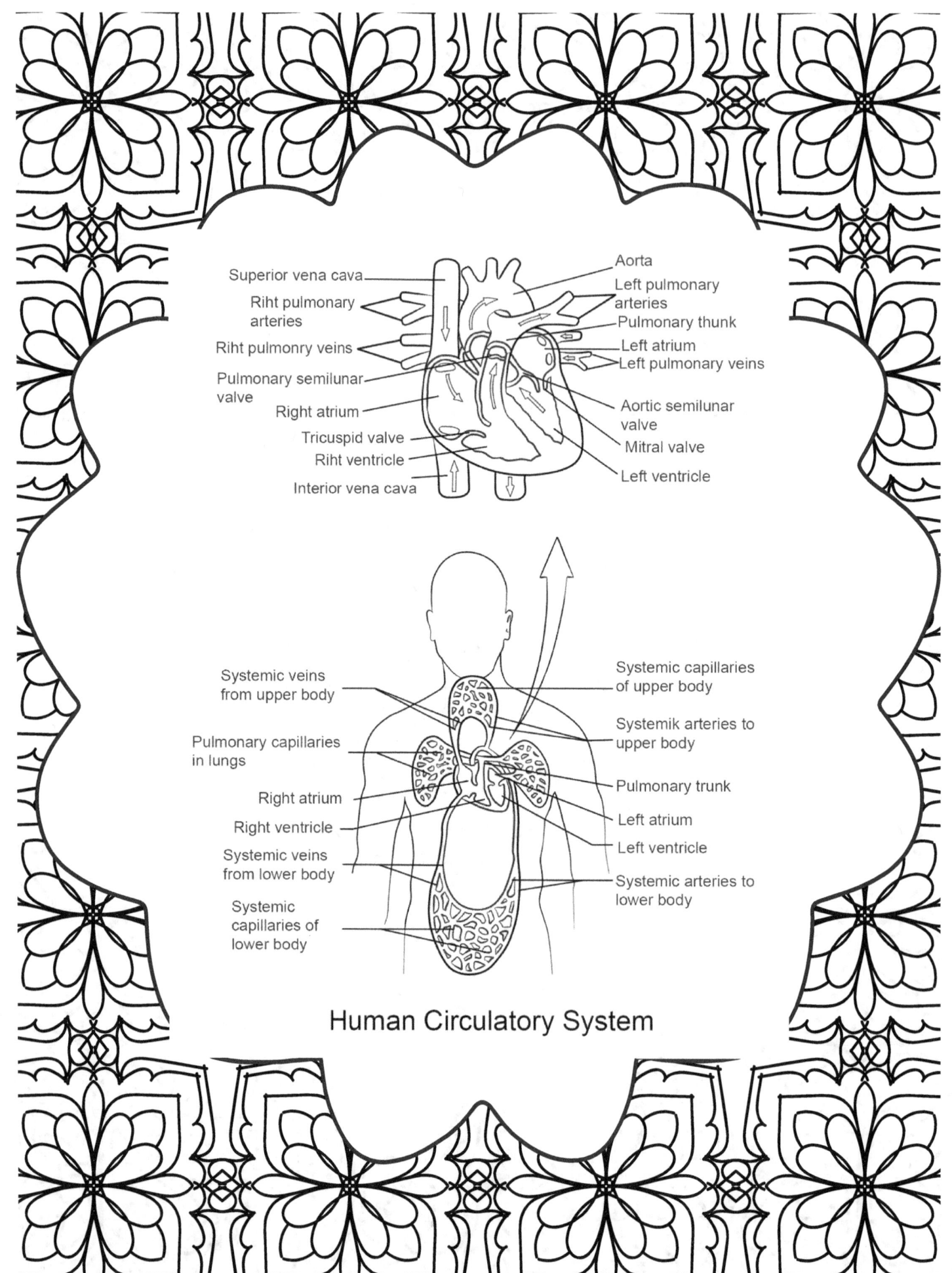

Superior vena cava

Riht pulmonary
arteries

Riht pulmonry veins

Pulmonary semilunar
valve

Right atrium

Tricuspid valve

Riht ventricle

Interior vena cava

Aorta

Left pulmonary
arteries

Pulmonary thunk

Left atrium

Left pulmonary veins

Aortic semilunar
valve

Mitral valve

Left ventricle

Systemic veins
from upper body

Pulmonary capillaries
in lungs

Right atrium

Right ventricle

Systemic veins
from lower body

Systemic
capillaries of
lower body

Systemic capillaries
of upper body

Systemik arteries to
upper body

Pulmonary trunk

Left atrium

Left ventricle

Systemic arteries to
lower body

Human Circulatory System

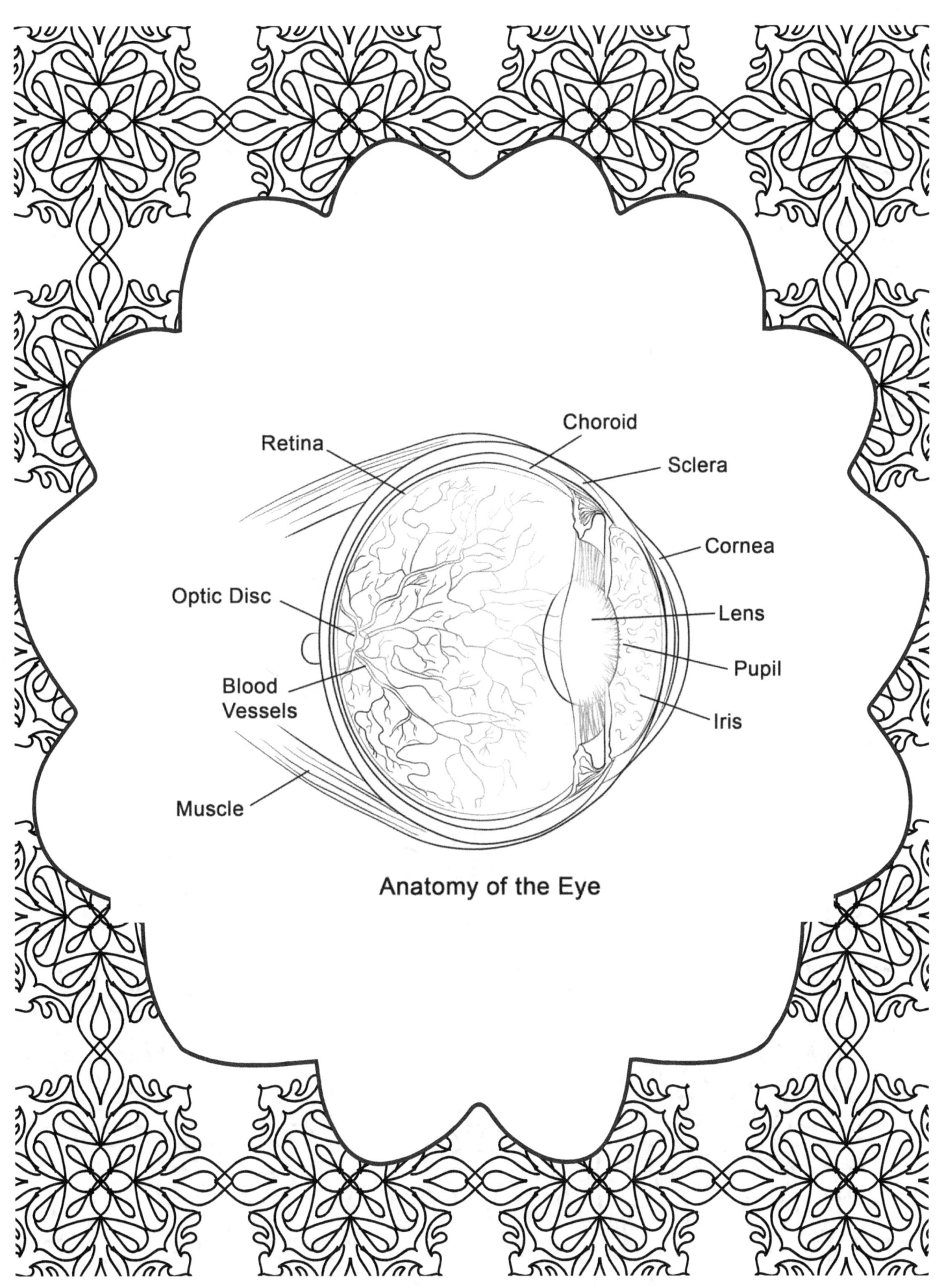

Anatomy of the Eye

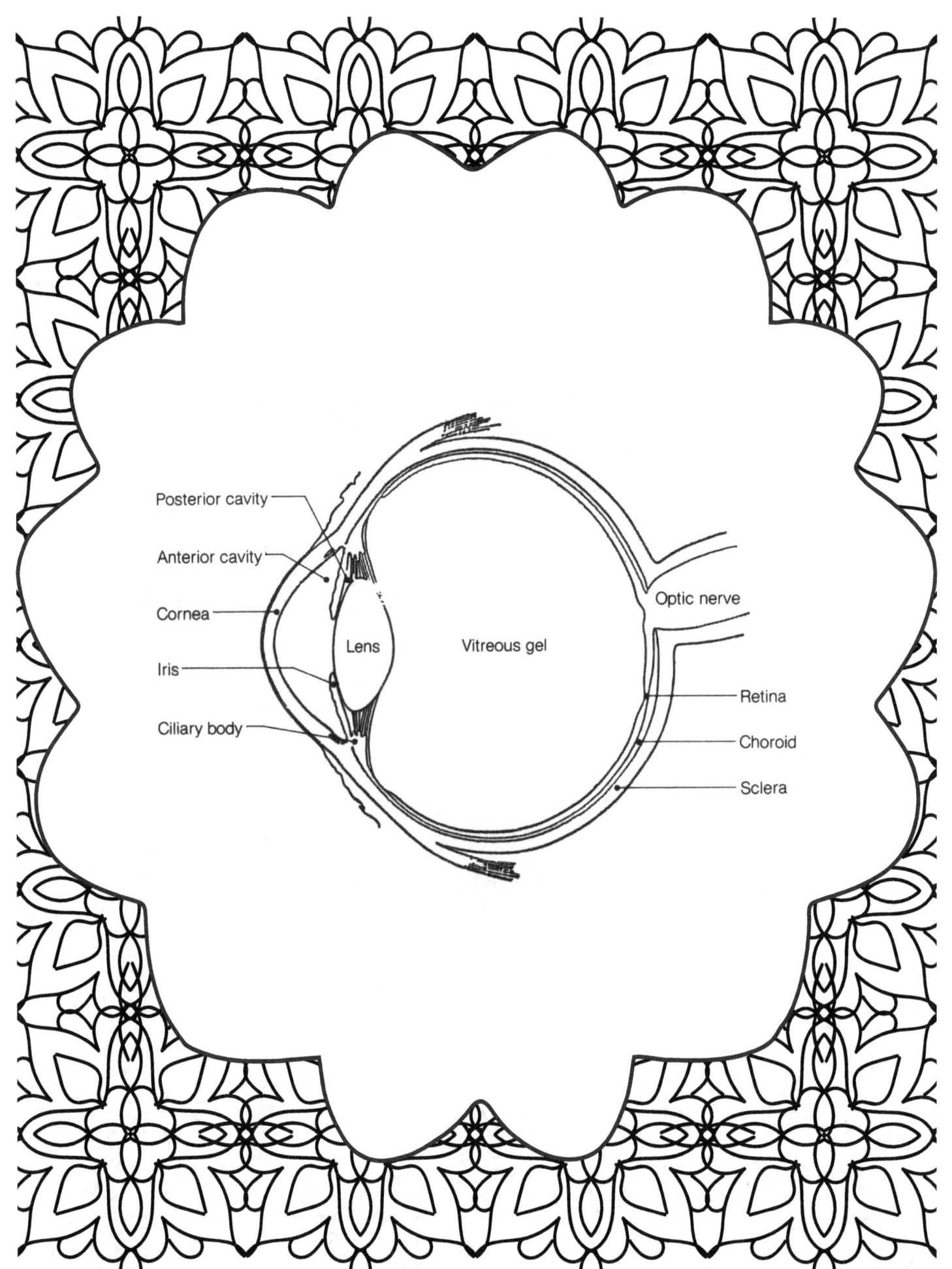

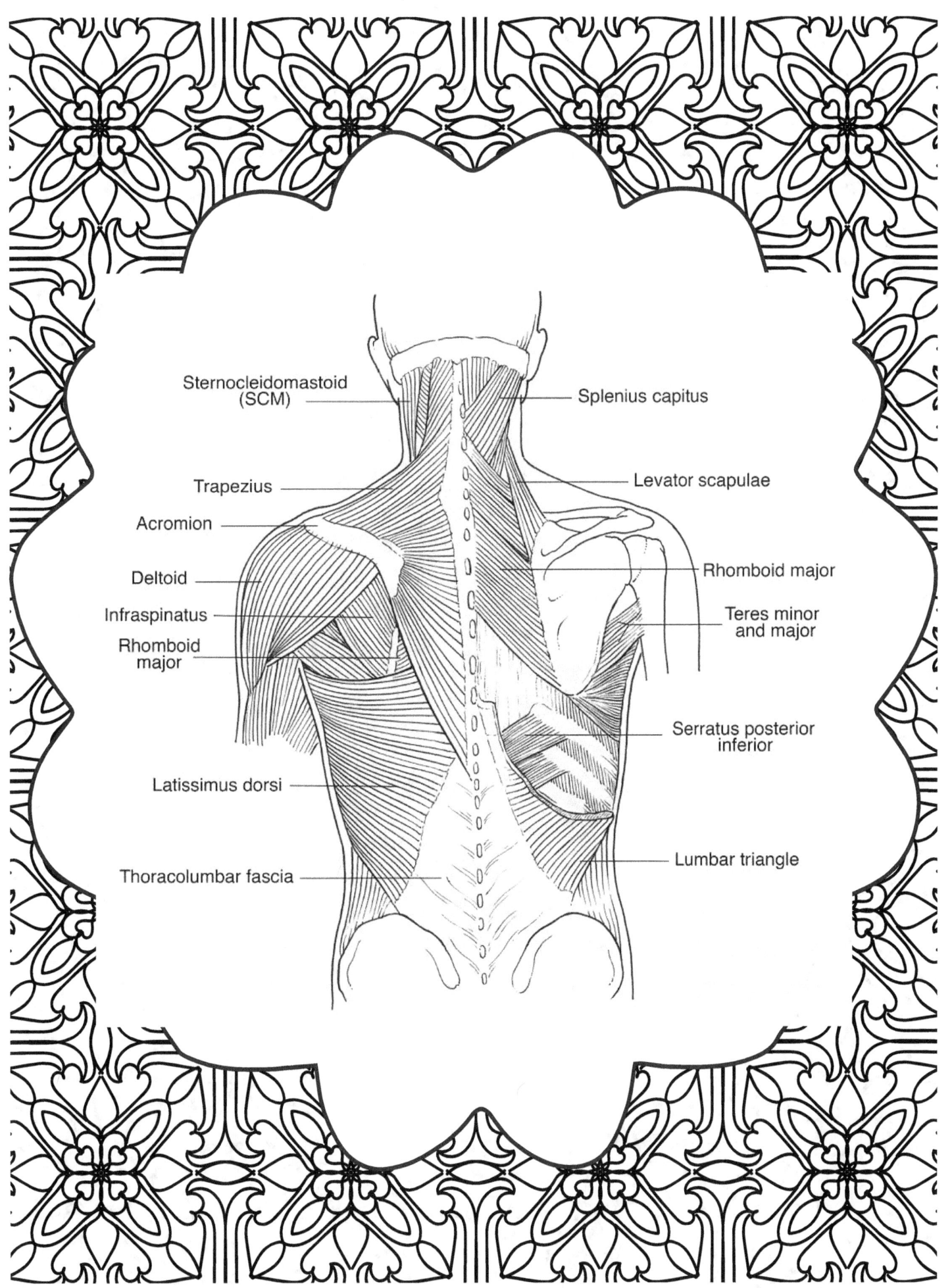

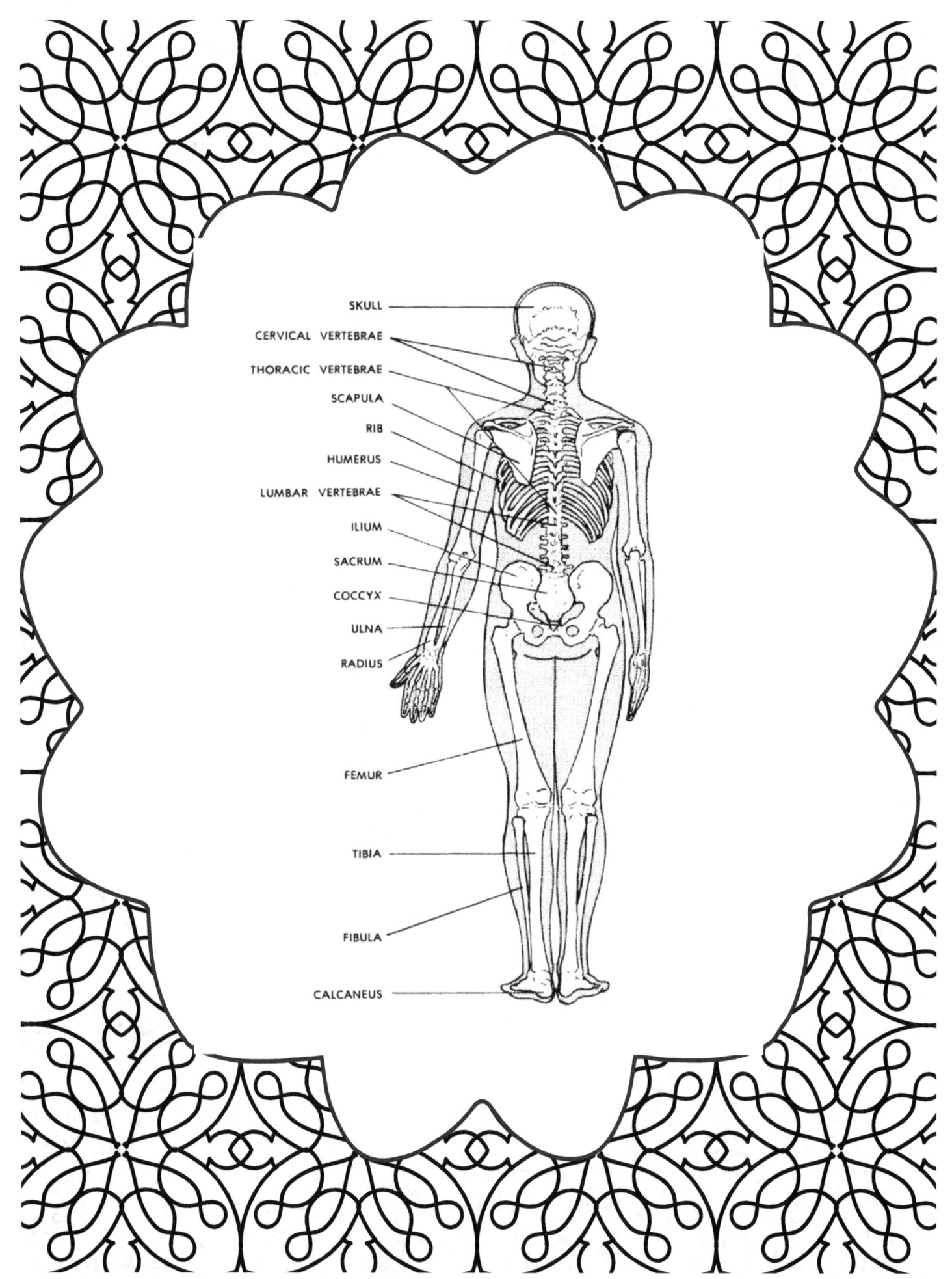

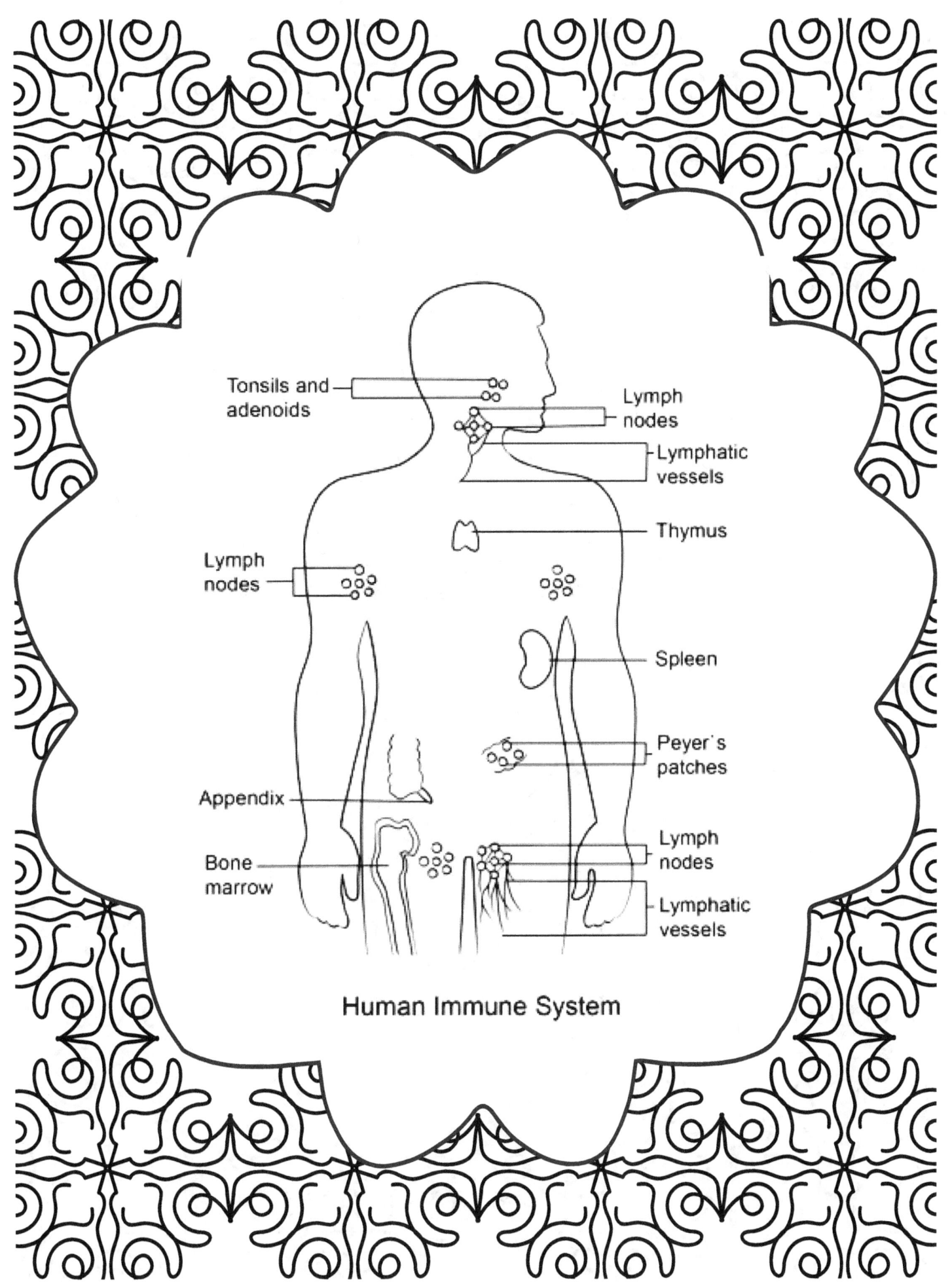

Human Immune System

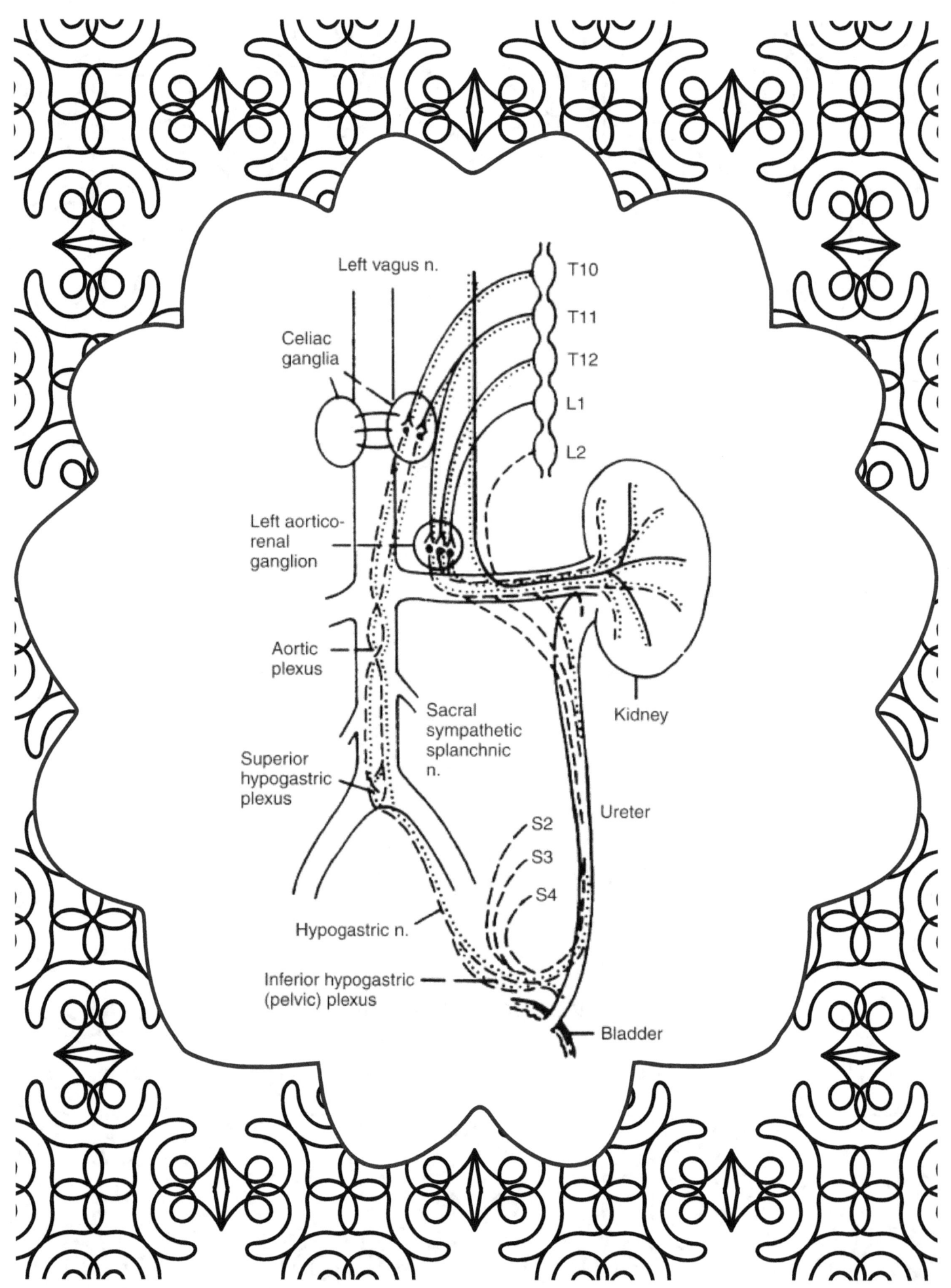

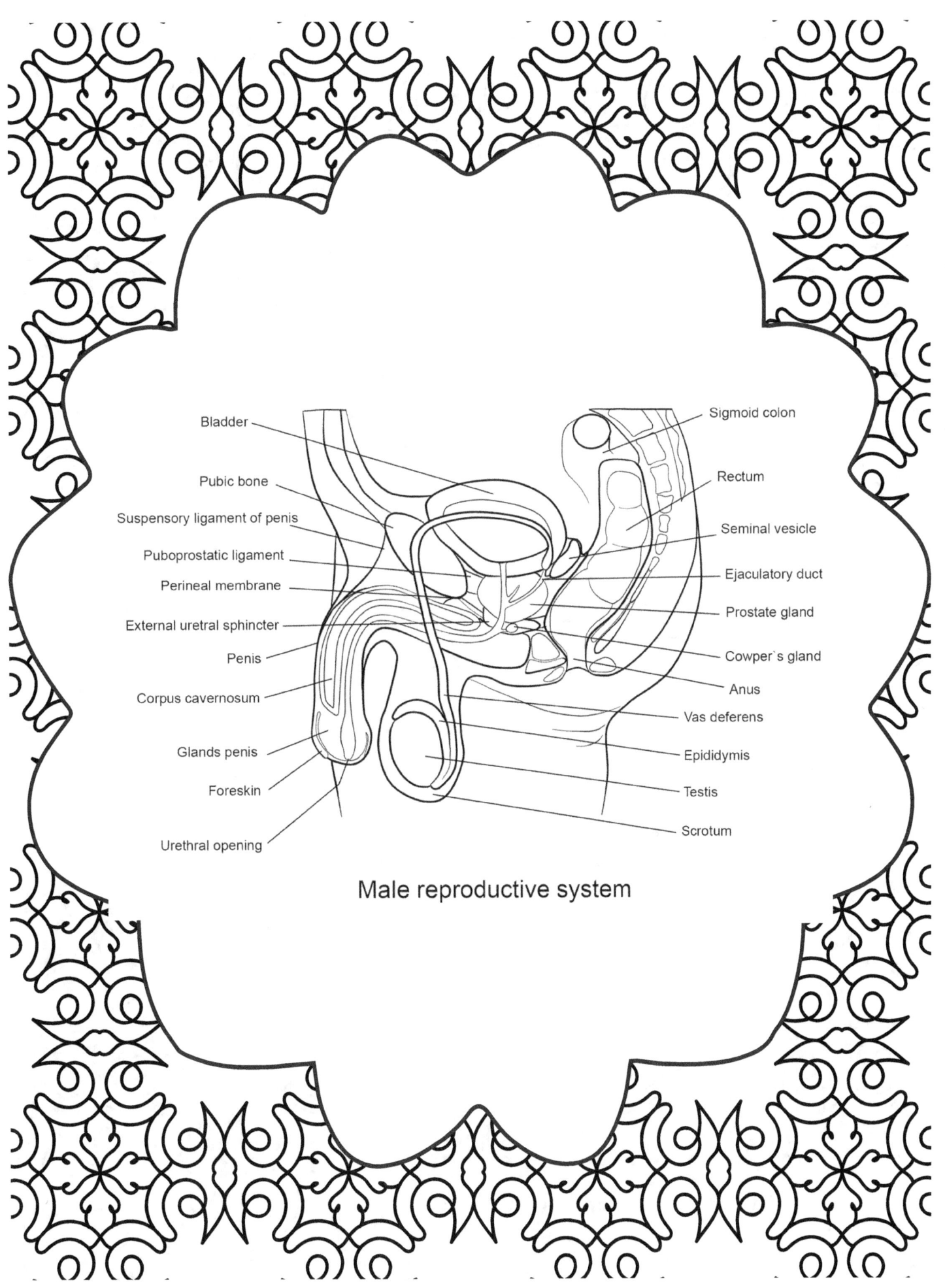

Male reproductive system

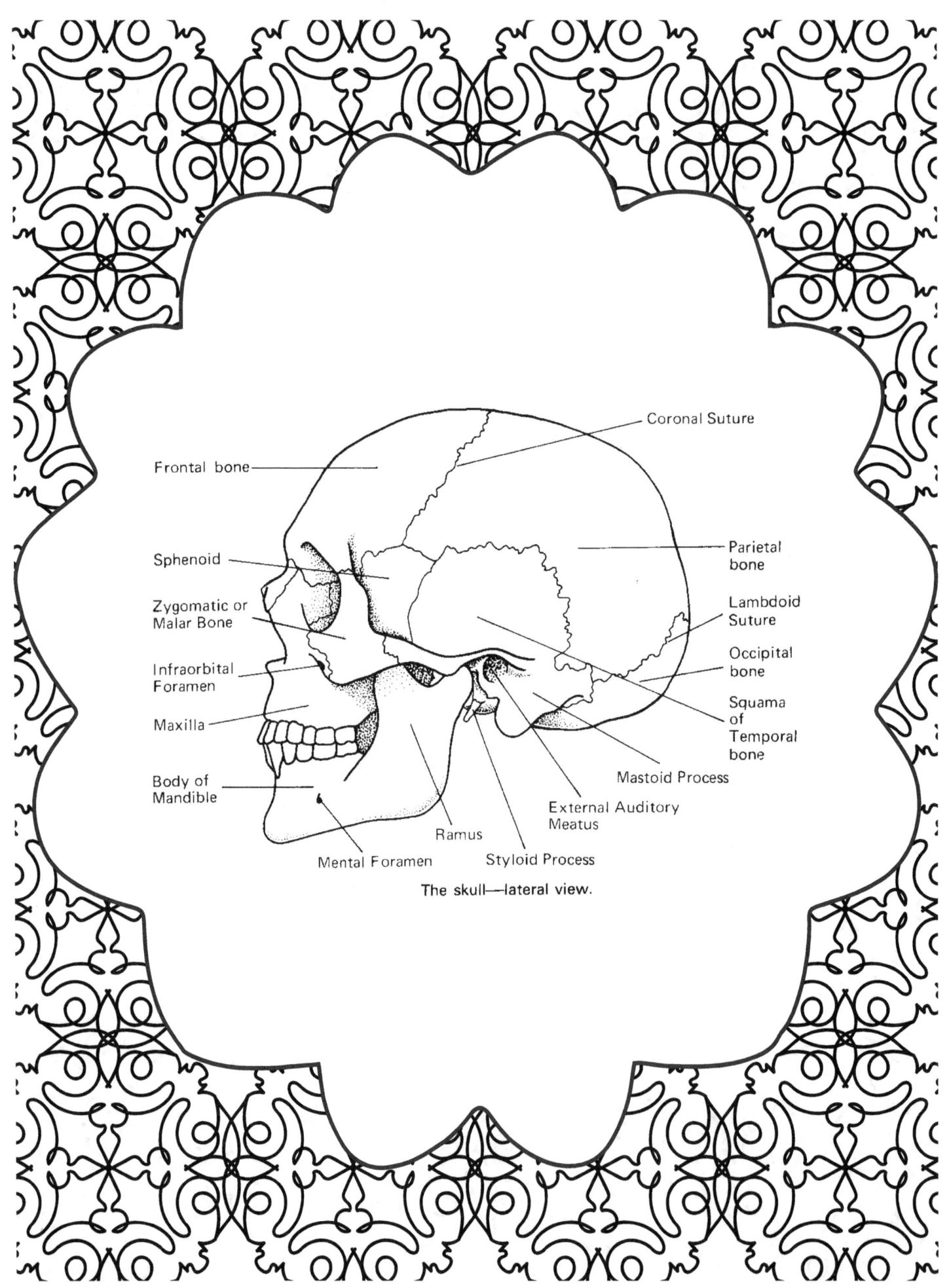

The skull—lateral view.

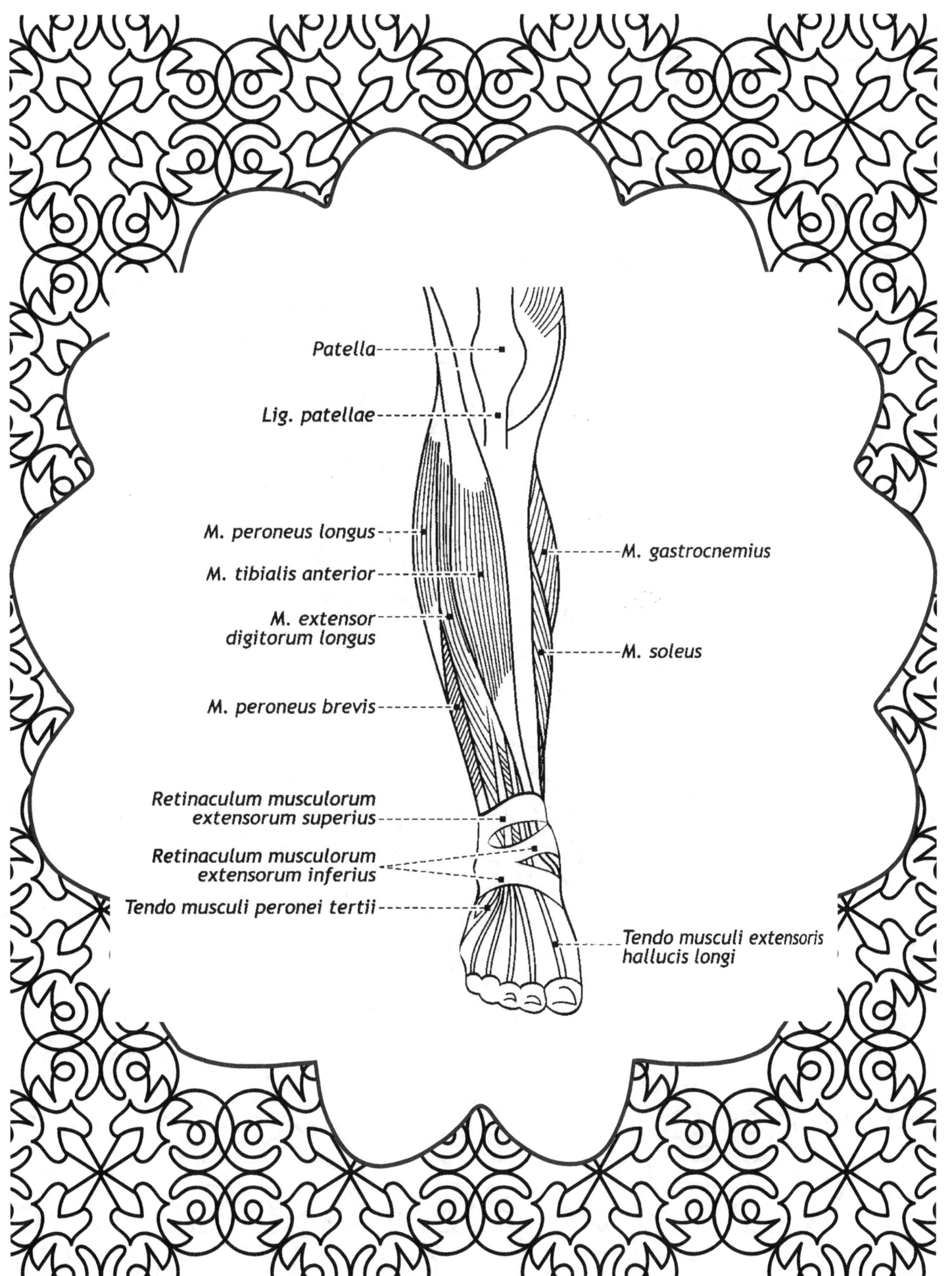

Patella

Lig. patellae

M. peroneus longus

M. tibialis anterior

M. extensor
digitorum longus

M. peroneus brevis

Retinaculum musculorum
extensorum superius

Retinaculum musculorum
extensorum inferius

Tendo musculi peronei tertii

M. gastrocnemius

M. soleus

Tendo musculi extensoris
hallucis longi

Color the Bony Features of the Pelvis

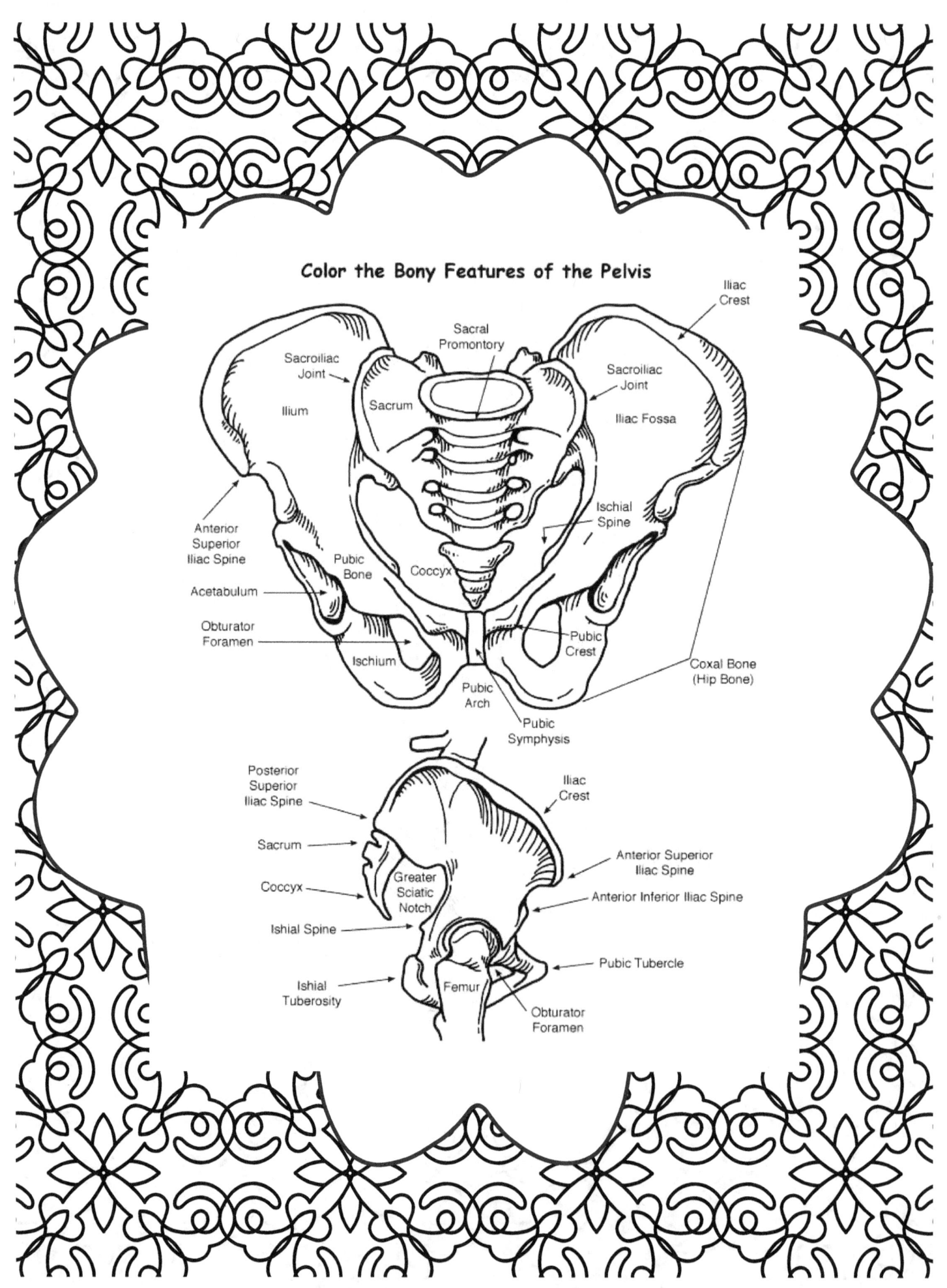

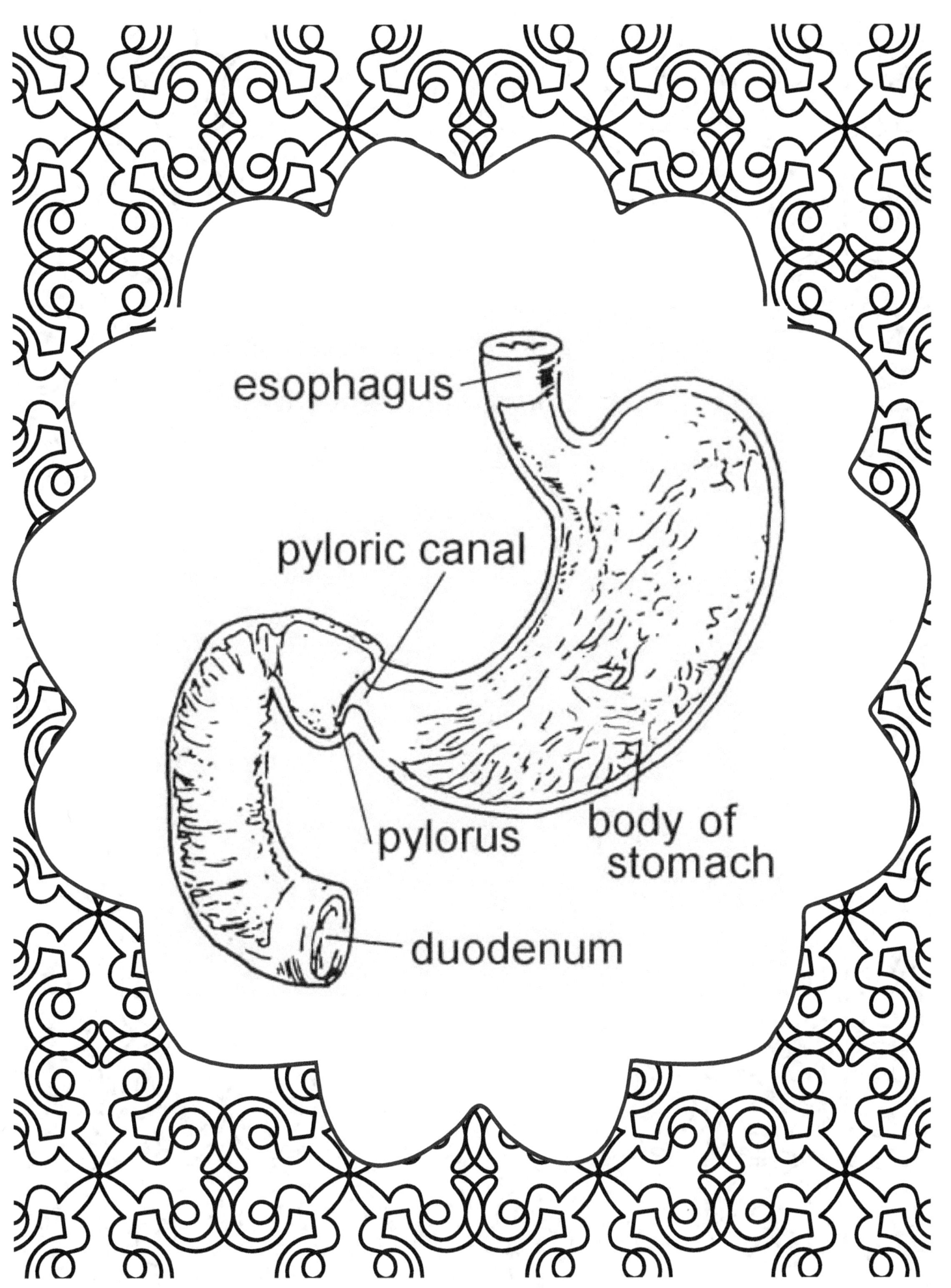

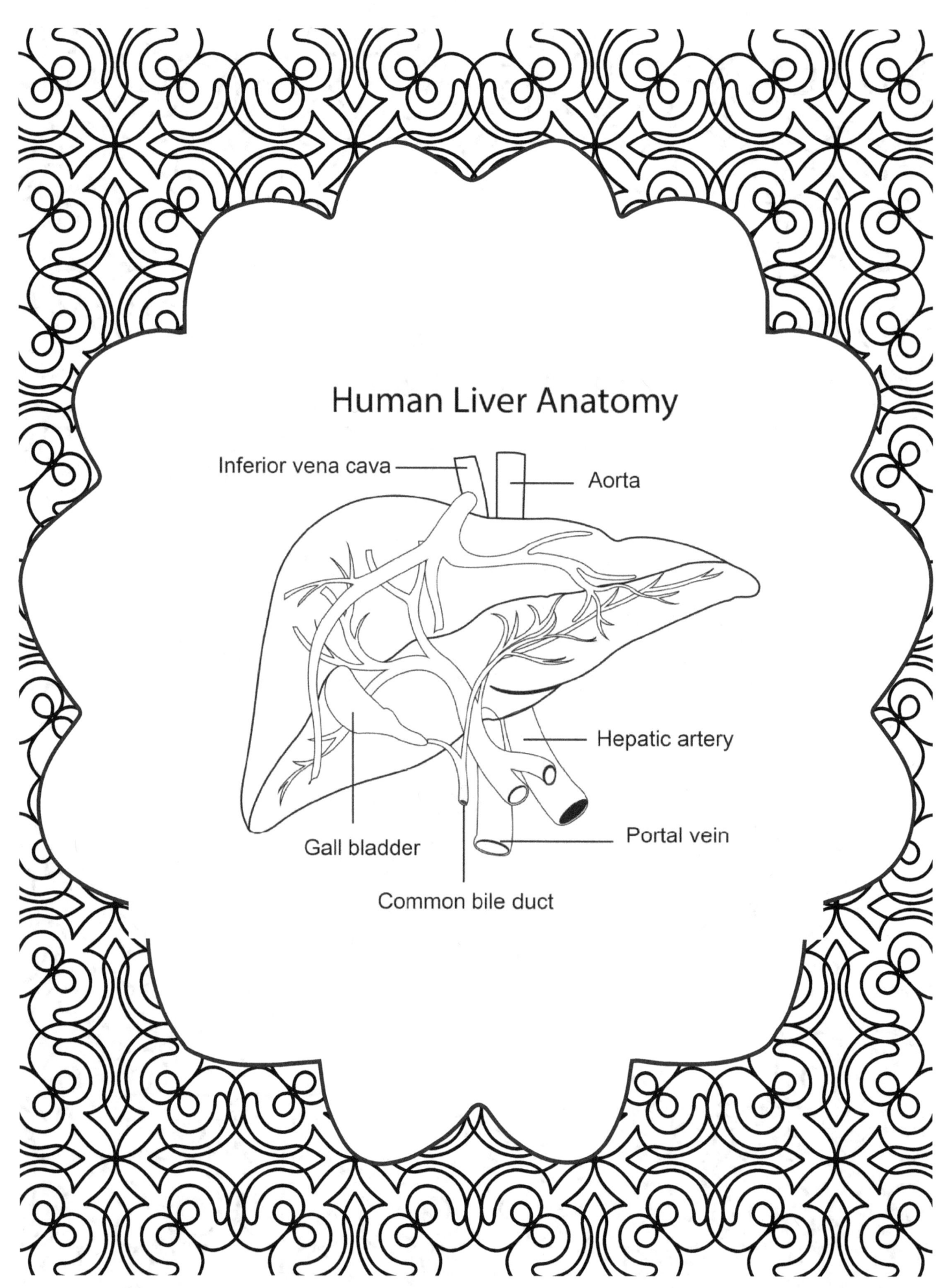

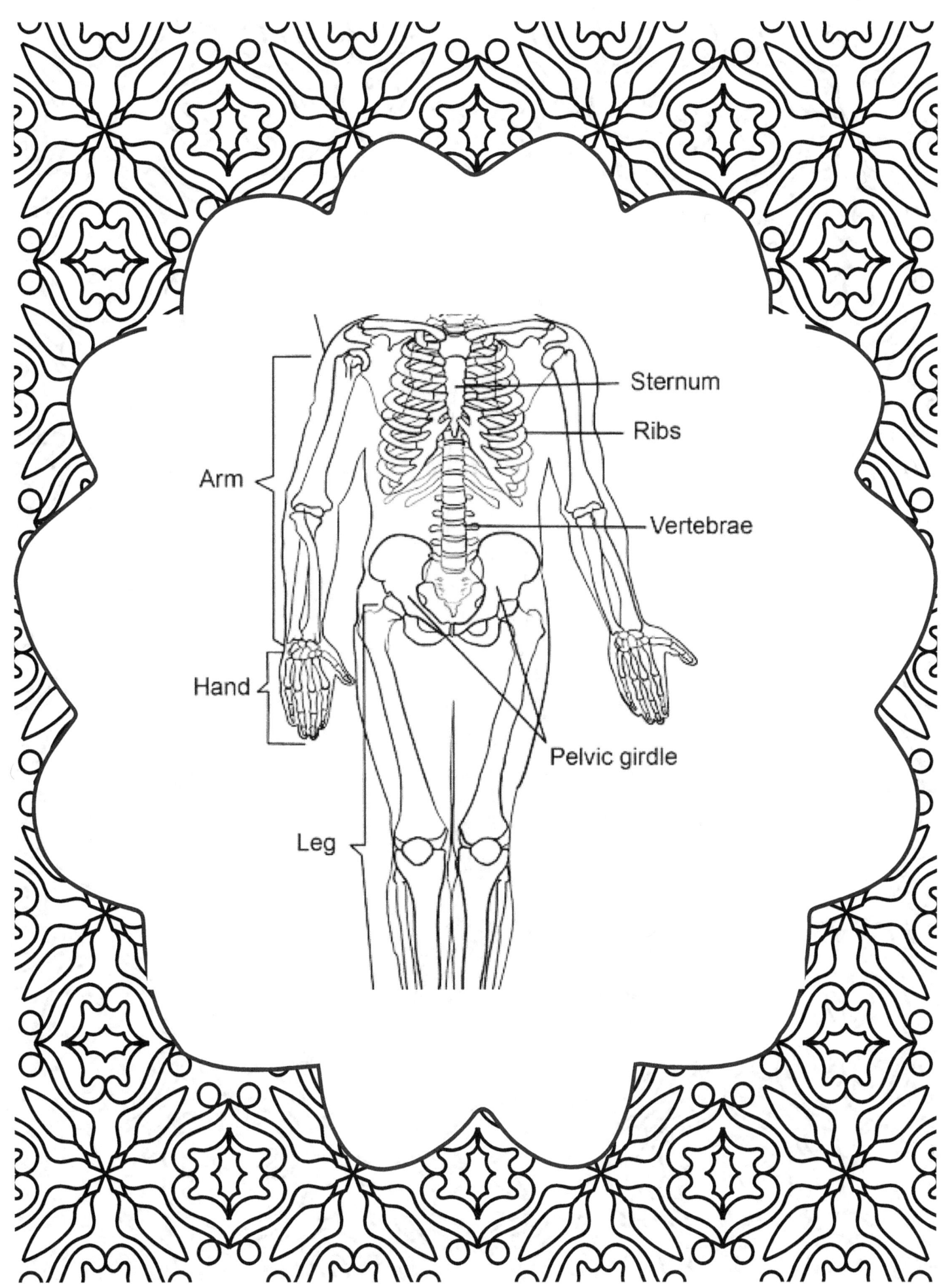

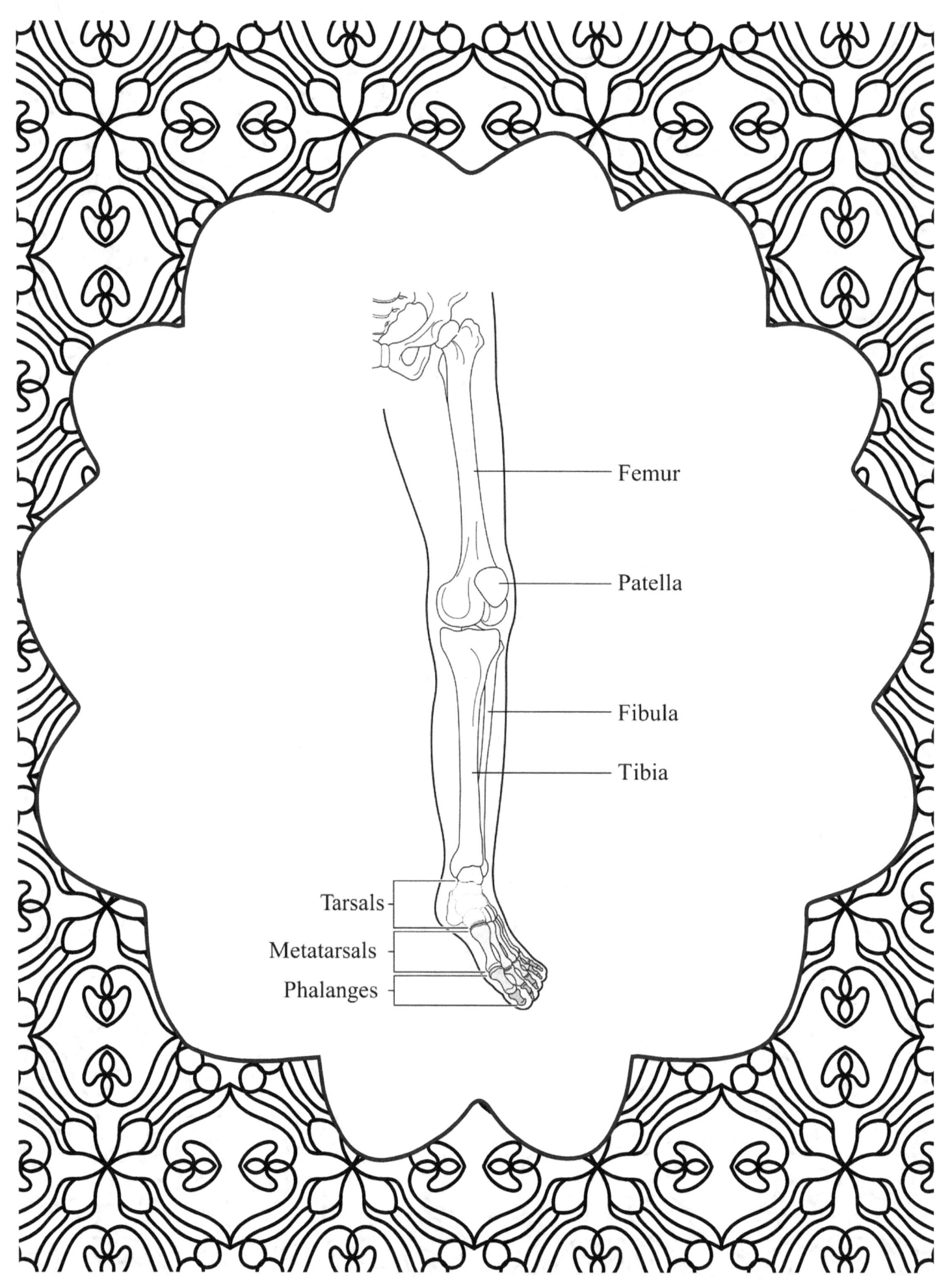

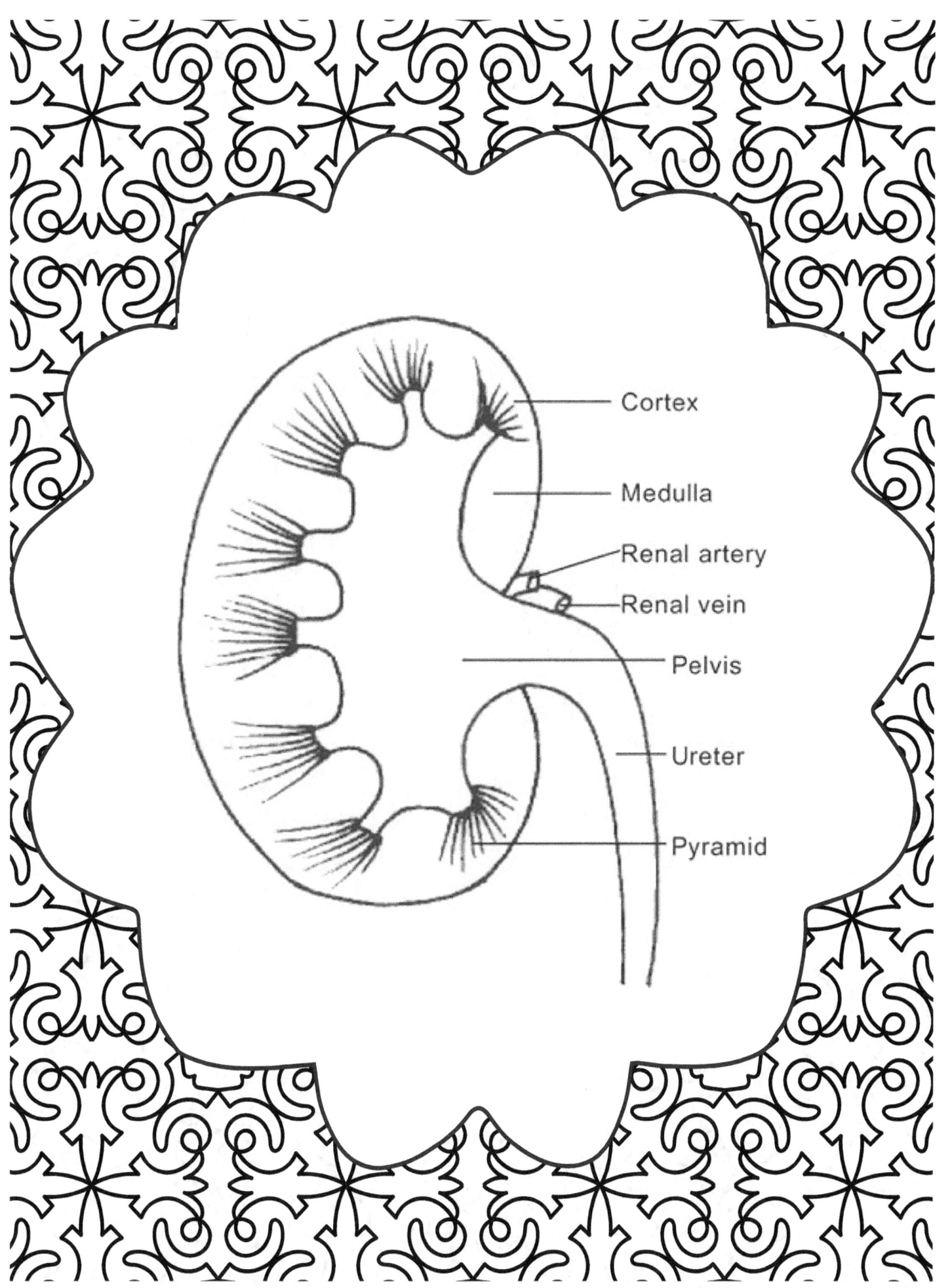

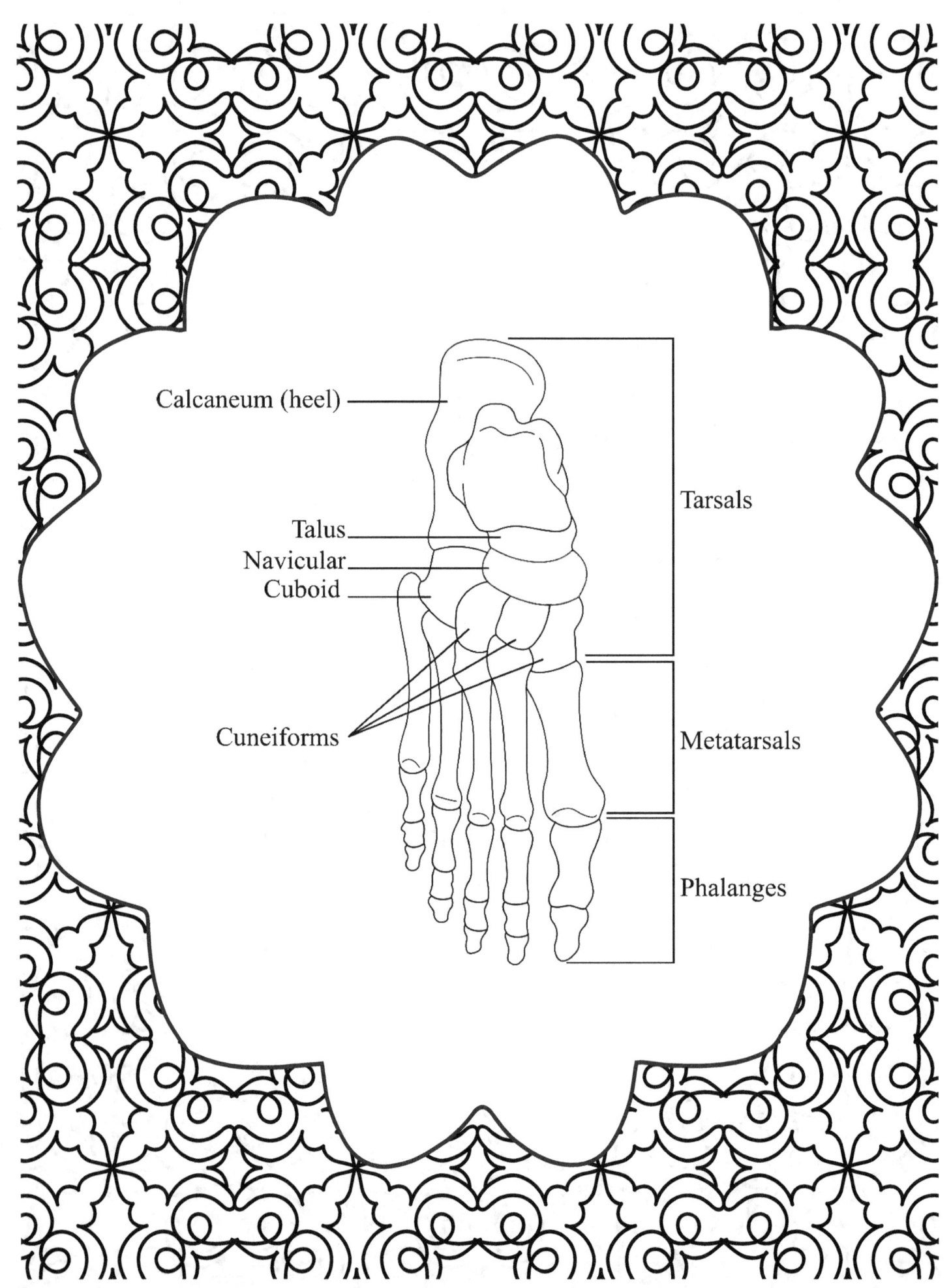

Calcaneum (heel)

Talus
Navicular
Cuboid

Cuneiforms

Tarsals

Metatarsals

Phalanges

Color the Arteries of the Head and Neck

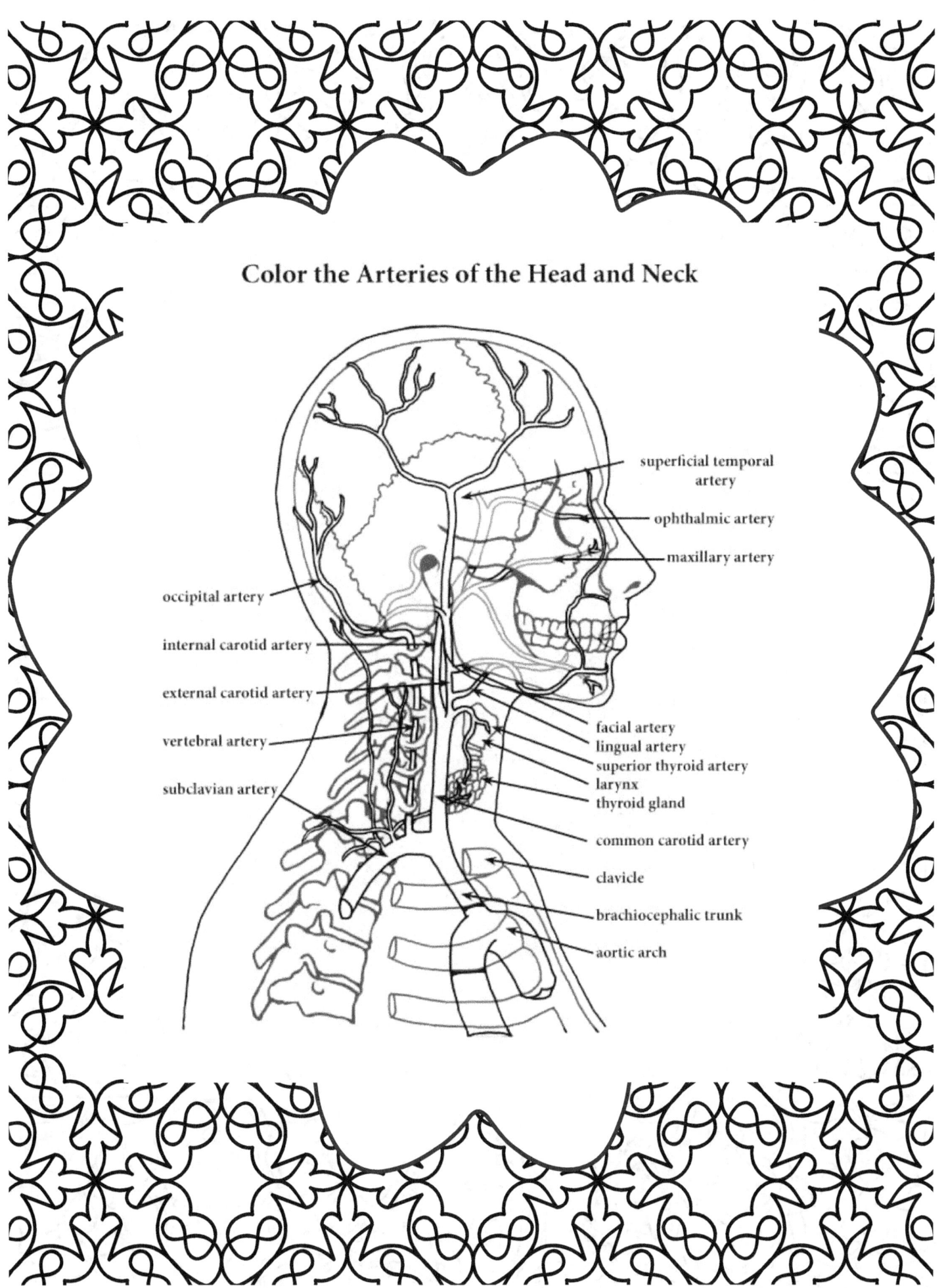

superficial temporal artery

ophthalmic artery

maxillary artery

occipital artery

internal carotid artery

external carotid artery

vertebral artery

subclavian artery

facial artery
lingual artery
superior thyroid artery
larynx
thyroid gland

common carotid artery

clavicle

brachiocephalic trunk

aortic arch

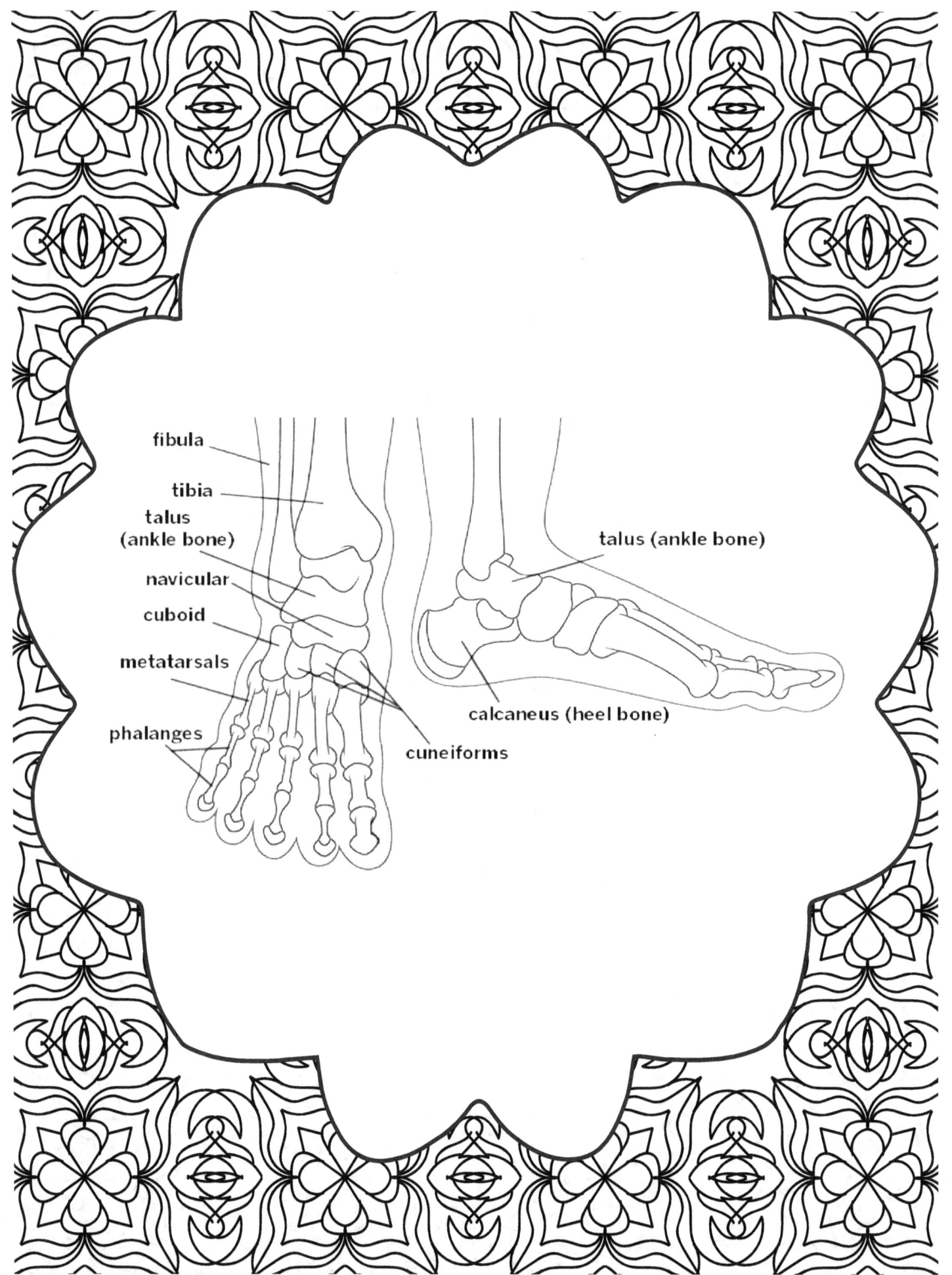

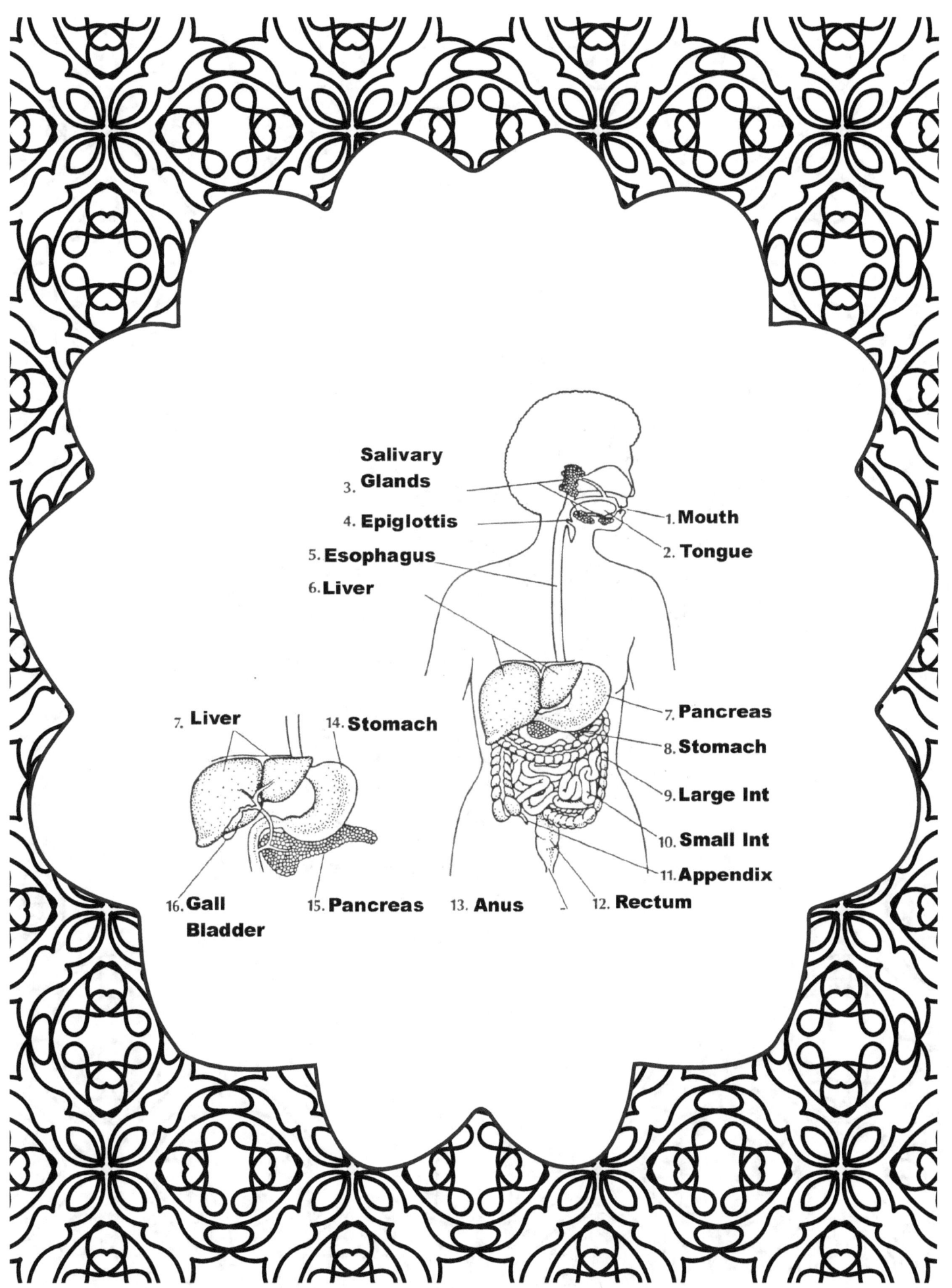

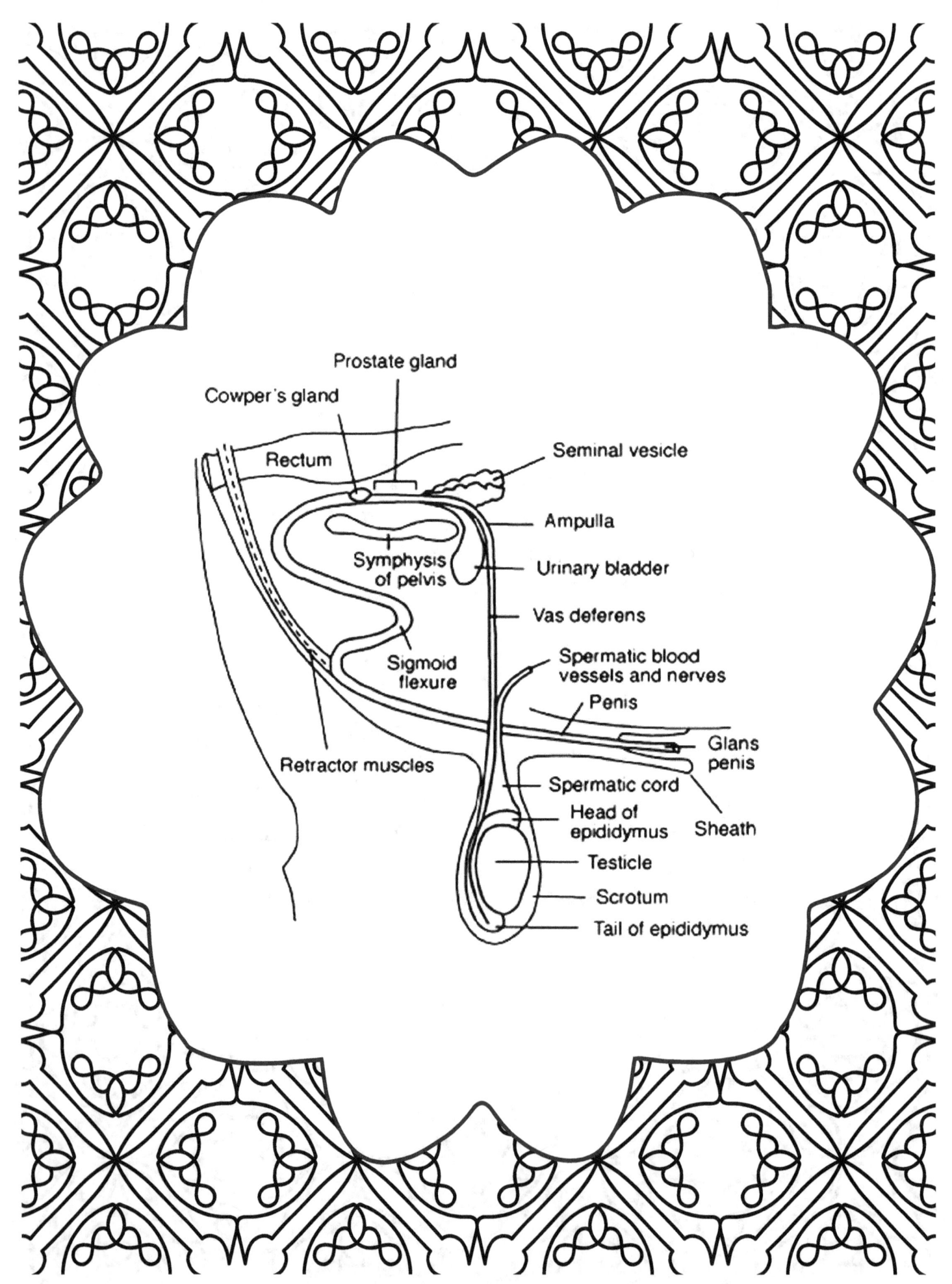

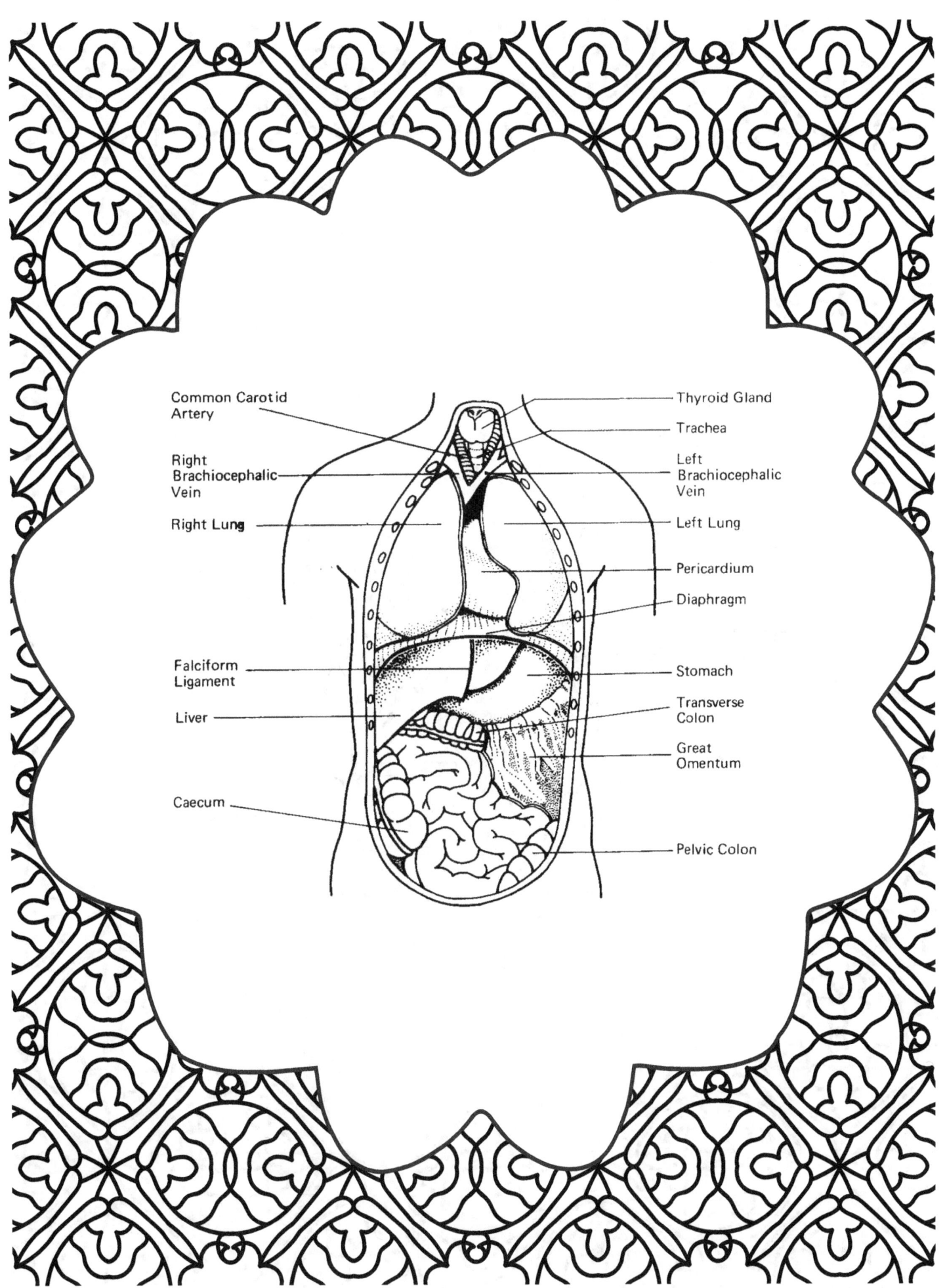

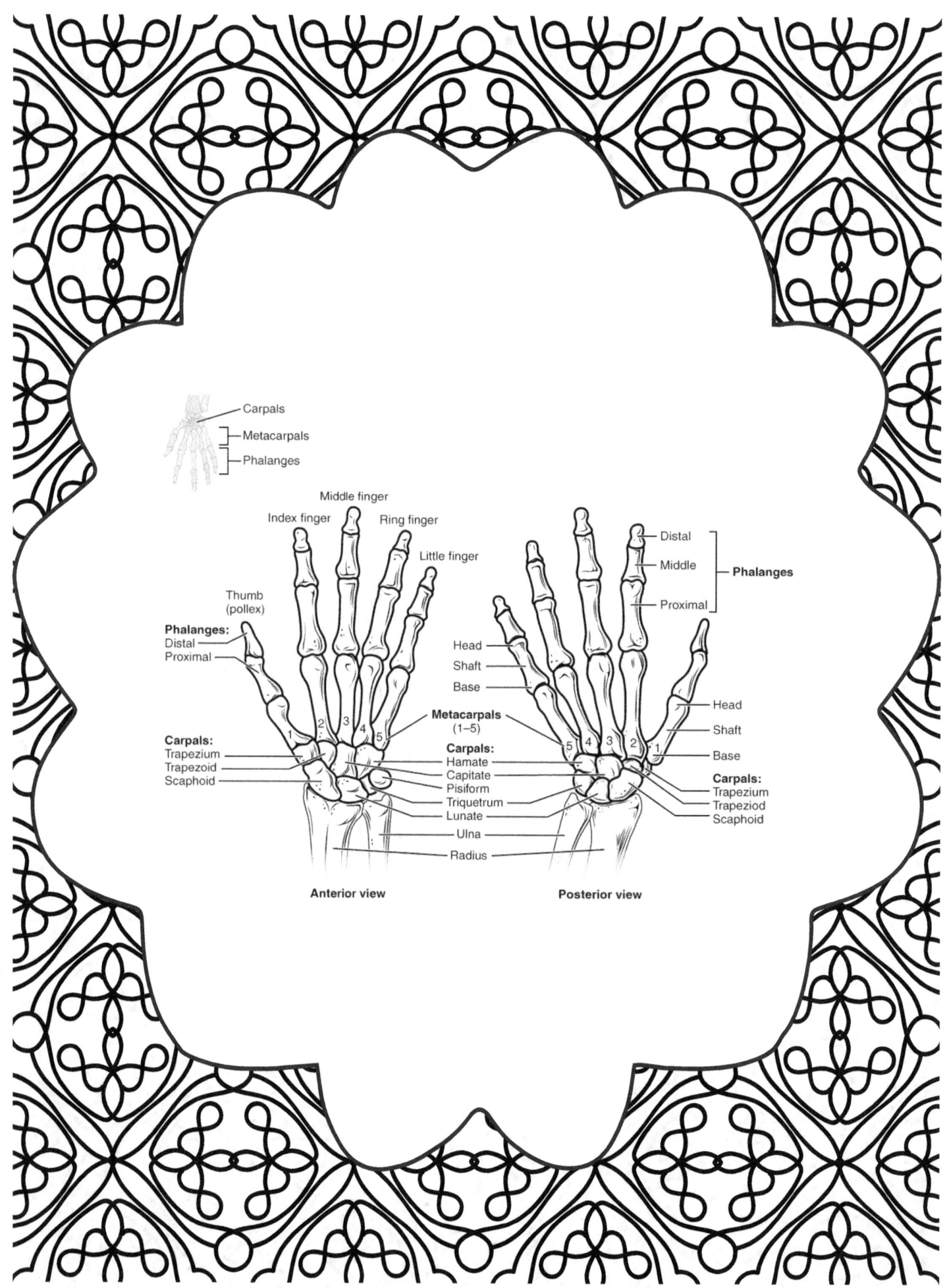

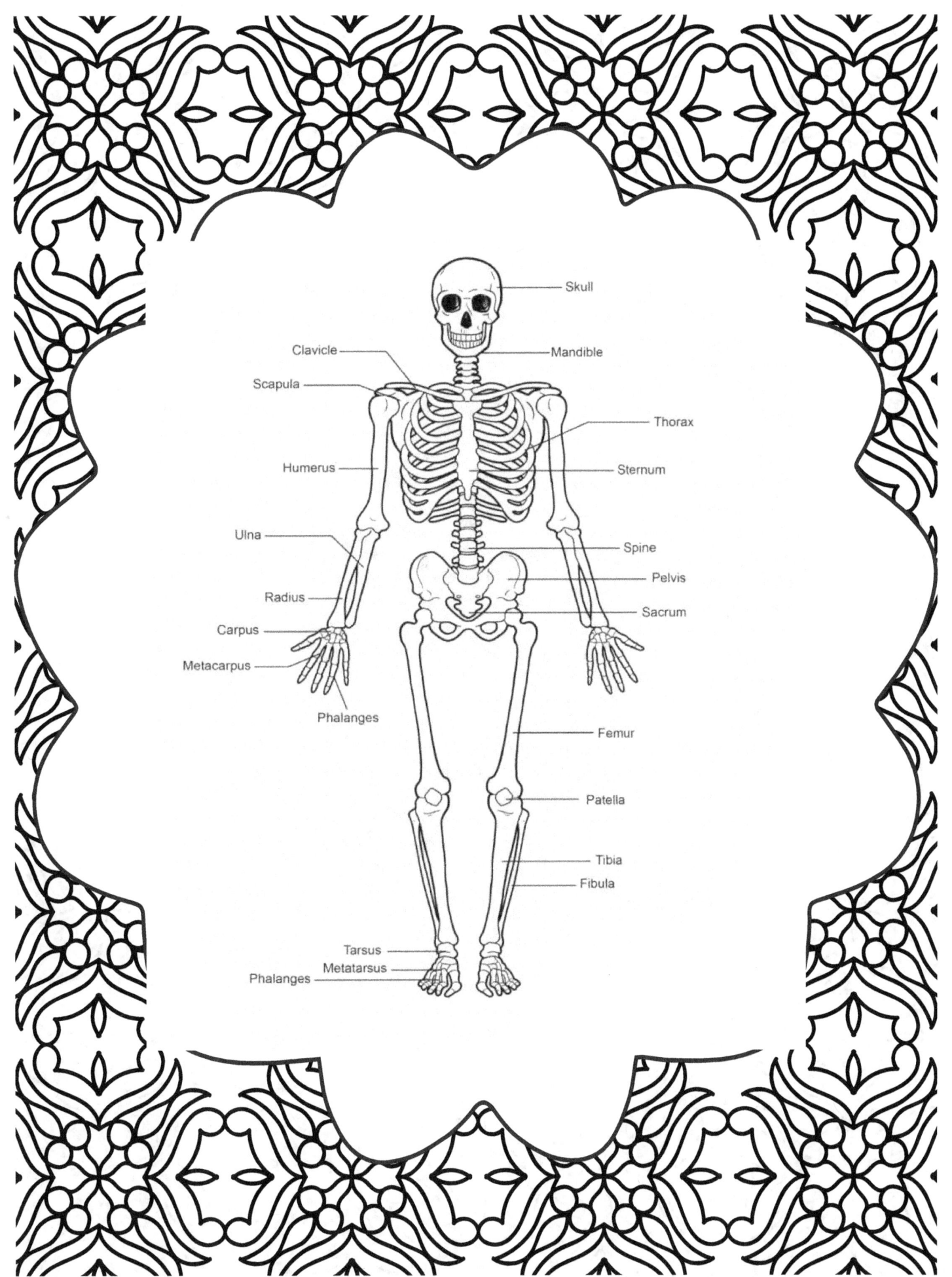

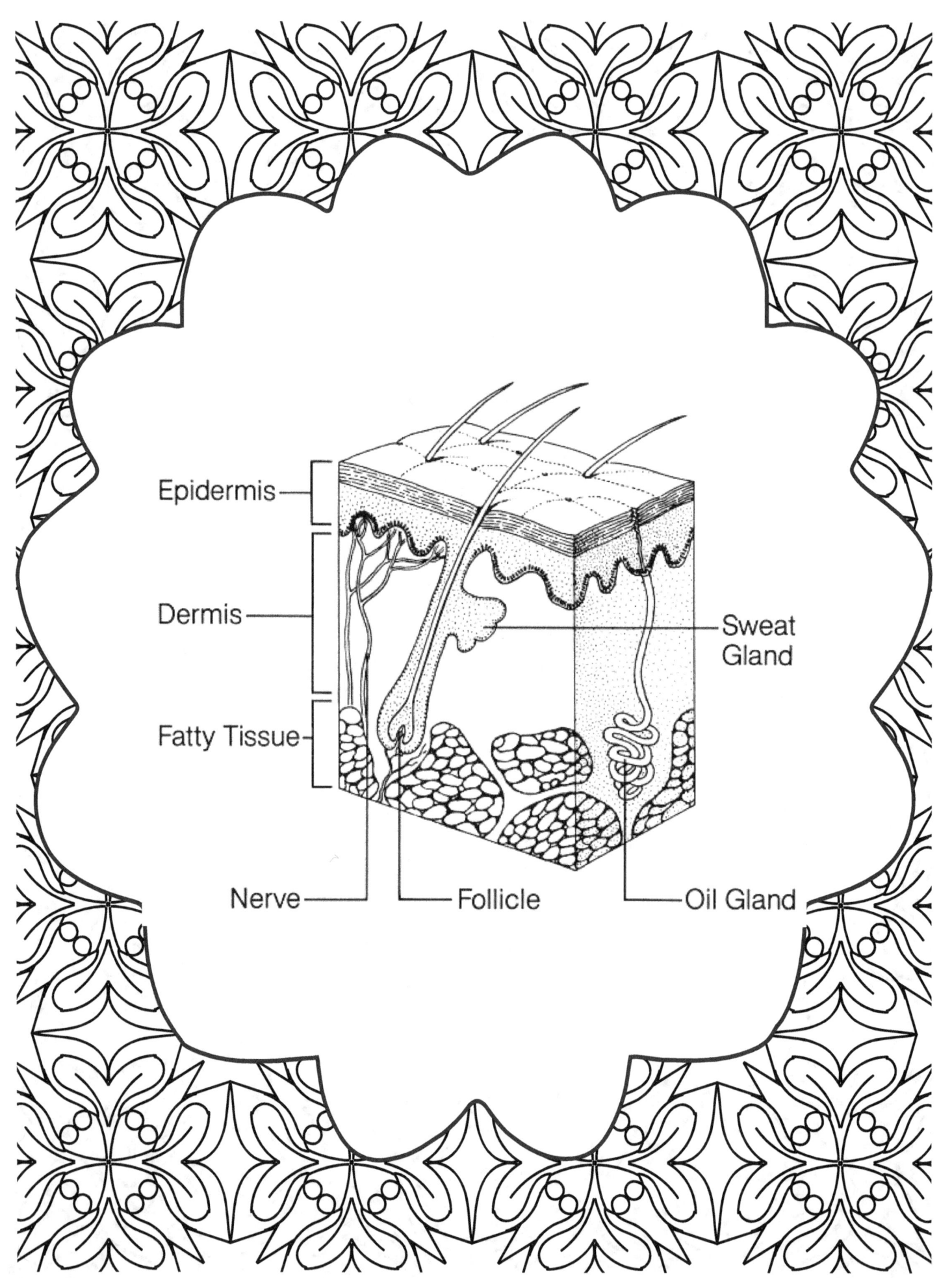

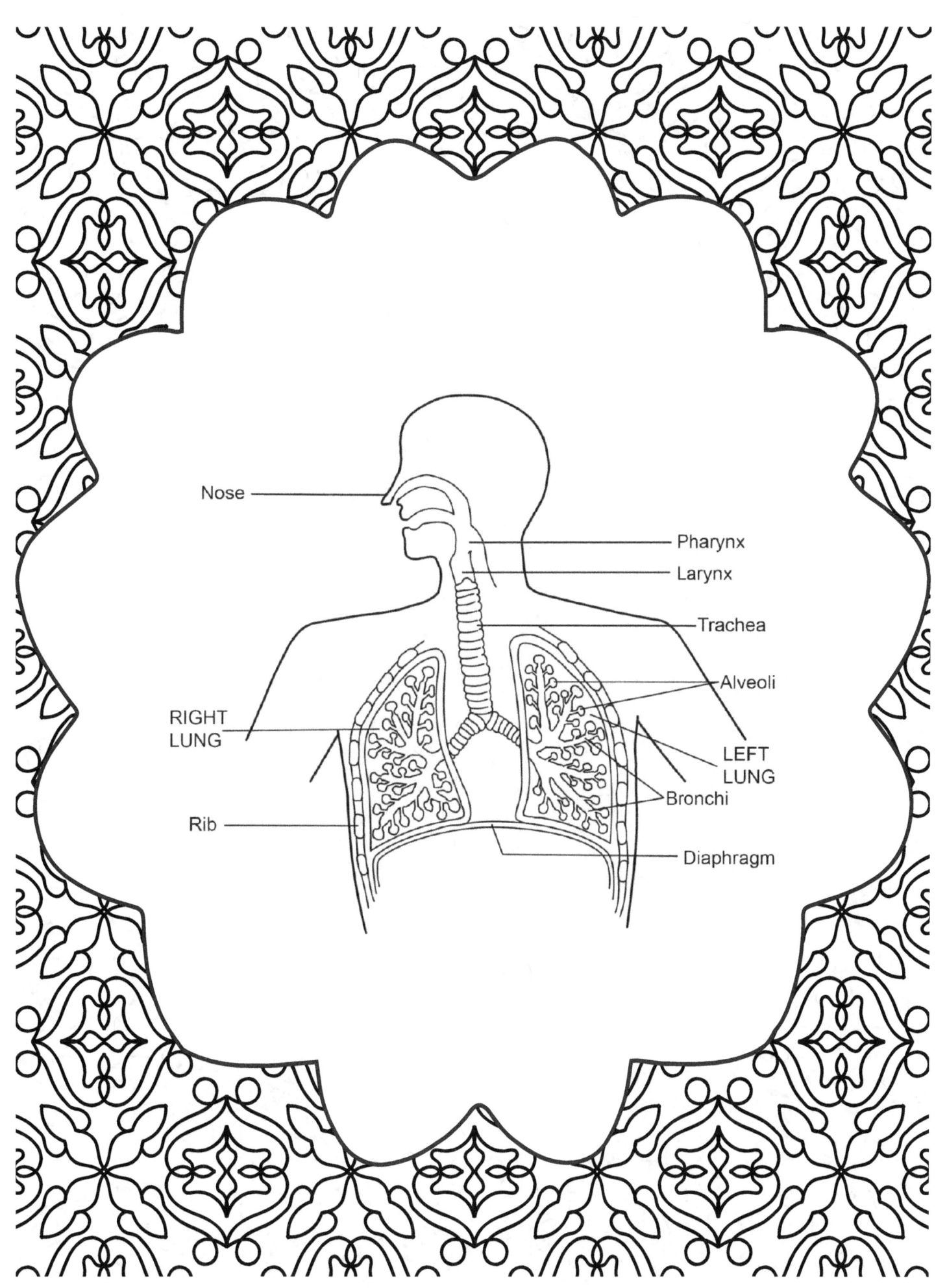

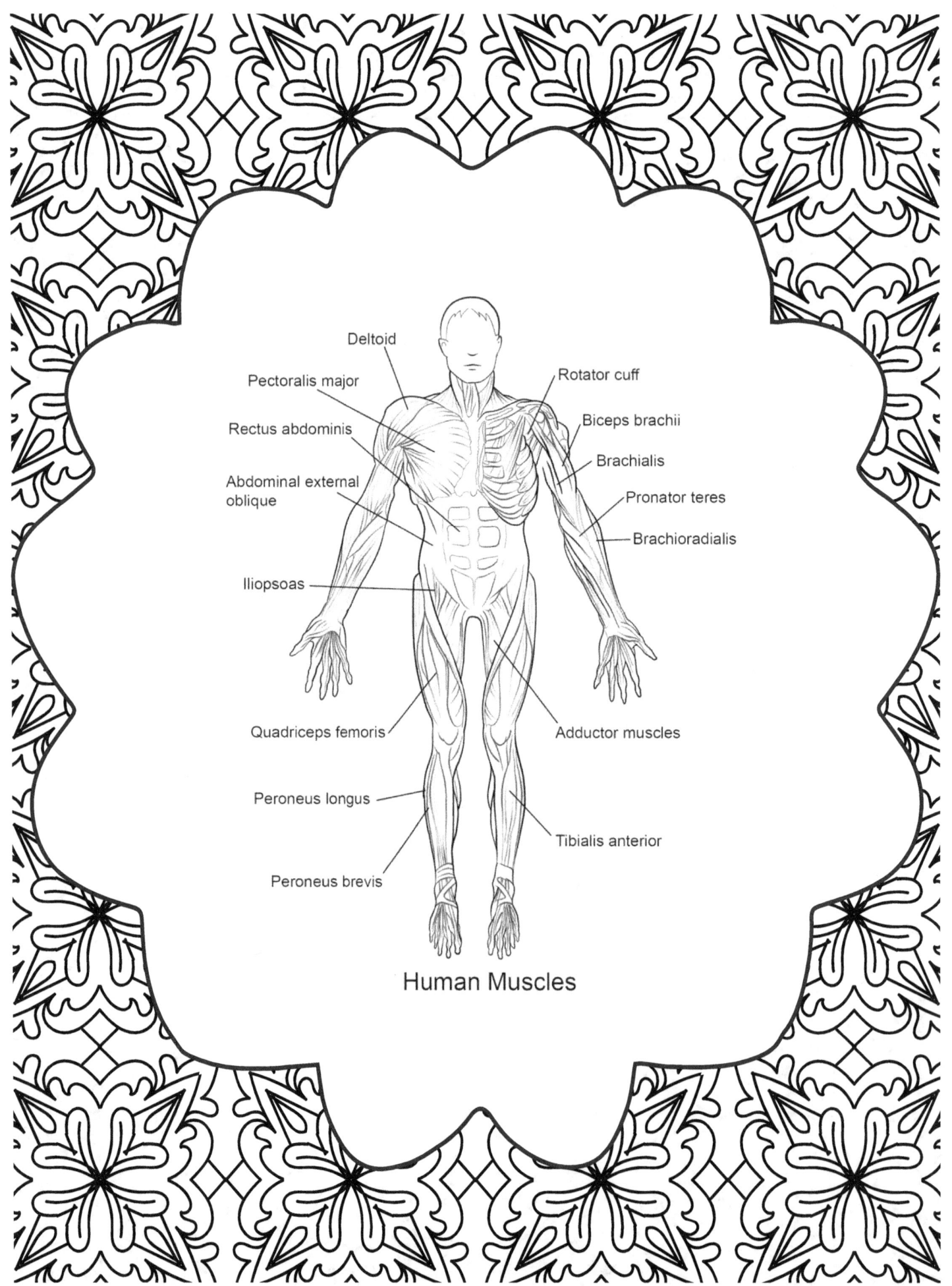

Human Muscles

www.ingramcontent.com/pod-product-compliance
Lightning Source LLC
Chambersburg PA
CBHW060006230526
45472CB00008B/1970